CLARE MAXWELL-HUDSON

AROMATHERAPY
MASSAGE

CLARE MAXWELL-HUDSON

AROMATHERAPY
MASSAGE

DORLING KINDERSLEY

LONDON • NEW YORK • SYDNEY

www.dk.com

A DORLING KINDERSLEY BOOK
www.dk.com

Massage Photography Sandra Lousada

Art Editor Jo Grey
Project Editor Helen Townsend
Designer Helen Diplock
D.T.P. Designer Karen Ruane

Senior Art Editor Tracy Timson
Senior Editor Susannah Marriott

Managing Art Editor Carole Ash
Managing Editor Rosie Pearson
Production Manager Maryann Rogers

This book is dedicated to my mother

2 4 6 8 10 9 7 5 3 1

A0033767
29.03.2001
7.99
646.75

First published in Great Britain in 1994 by
Dorling Kindersley Limited,
9 Henrietta Street, London WC2E 8PS

Second paperback edition 1999
Copyright © 1994, 1999
Dorling Kindersley Limited, London
Text copyright © 1994, 1999 Clare Maxwell-Hudson
Massage photography © 1994, 1999 Sandra Lousada

A CIP catalogue record for this book is available from
the British Library

ISBN 0 7513 0740 8

Reproduced by Colourscan, Singapore
Printed and bound in Singapore
by Star Standard Industries (Pte.) Ltd.

CONTENTS

INTRODUCTION

Fragrant essential oils can enrich your life, whether they are used therapeutically, in beauty treatments, to perfume the home or for sheer pleasure. But when the oils are combined with massage their effectiveness in relieving stress, improving mood and promoting good health is most striking.

What is Aromatherapy?

"Aroma" derives from the Greek word for spice – today we use the word more broadly to mean fragrance – and "therapy" means treatment, so aromatherapy literally means curative treatment by the use of scent. My research into the therapeutic properties of essential oils and the plants from which they derive has led me all over the world and brought me into contact with many cultures in which essential oils are valued. In *Aromatherapy Massage,* I reveal the traditional healing qualities attributed to my favourite oils and discuss the properties ascribed to them by the latest research. I have always added essential oils to oil blends in the belief that they enhance the effects of a massage. Odours are perceived by the part of the brain connected with emotion, so a pleasurable scent can have a positive effect on your enjoyment of life.

The Art of Massage

Massage is probably the oldest and simplest of medical treatments. Rubbing an aching shoulder or soothing a furrowed brow is a healing instinct common to all cultures. Over two thousand years ago, the Greek physician Hippocrates said "rubbing can bind a joint that is too loose and loosen a joint that is too rigid". This is the most fascinating part of massage: the same strokes can produce so many different effects. Brisk movements invigorate, while similar movements performed slowly can induce sleep. And, because massage is almost second nature, the techniques are easy to learn. The physical benefits of massage, such as improved circulation and relaxed muscles, and the psychological feelings of being comforted and cared for, produce a sense of well-being which is surely unique.

TOUCH & SCENT

Aromatherapy massage is an art that operates through the empathy between the person giving the massage, the person receiving it and the aroma of the oils. Each blend of oils is individual, determined by the scents the recipient prefers and by their desired effect, whether it is to relieve minor ailments, to pamper with an aromatic beauty treatment, or simply to ease tension with a full body massage.

Over 700 years ago, Rumi, an Afghan poet and philosopher, related the benefits of aromatherapy in this story: Once upon a time, there was a man who had an illness which none seemed able to cure. After much travelling, he found a very wise doctor, who gave him a stick and told him to go for a walk with it every day. A month later, the man was completely cured. He returned to the doctor, who revealed that the handle of the stick was filled with aromatic plants and spices, and the heat and rubbing of the man's hand released their healing properties. I hope that aromatherapy will have the same beneficial effect for you and that *Aromatherapy Massage* will help you to experience touch and smell in the most pleasurable way through giving and receiving massage with scented oils.

Clare Maxwell-Hudson

ESSENTIAL OILS

*These concentrated essences extracted from plants
have been valued throughout history for their
therapeutic properties, and here I present over 20 of
my favourites. After a massage with a blend of
essential oils, a client captured their wonder,
"I was engulfed in aromatic oils. I had such an
incredible feeling of well-being and relaxation".*

AROMATHERAPY IN HISTORY

Many powers have been attributed to fragrant plants, and they have been used throughout history in the pursuit of happiness and health as part of medicine, religion, magic and cosmetics. In early civilizations, scented woods and oils were burned to communicate with gods or to exorcize demons, and incense still features in religious ceremonies. Massage with aromatic oils has also been used to soften and perfume the skin and to promote healing.

MASTER PERFUMERS

The Ancient Egyptians greatly appreciated fragrance, and wealthy men and women used scented oils daily in massage to soften and protect their skin from the harsh, dry climate. Cleopatra is even said to have seduced Mark Antony with fragrance, by covering the floors 46 centimetres (18 inches) deep in rose petals.

The Egyptians also used aromatic plants and oils to embalm the dead, demonstrating a sophisticated knowledge of their antiseptic properties. Ointments found in Tutankhamun's tomb, dating from *c.*1320BC, were found to contain frankincense, gum resins and spikenard, and remarkably, still retained their scent.

The Ancient Greeks learned about fragrance from the Egyptians, whom they revered as master perfumers. Believing aromatics enabled them to drink more wine, wealthy Athenians placed bags of fragrant flowers and vases of unguents on their banquet tables. Scented oils were also used for massage, and were thought to have medicinal properties – the lyric poet Anacreon (582–*c.*485BC) claimed "The best recipe for health is to apply sweet scents to the brain".

The Romans developed public baths believing in their health-giving properties, and bathing was followed by scented massage. Barbers soothed men's faces with hot towels and scented oils, and wealthy women refreshed their bodies with rose water. The knowledge of the healing properties of plants spread with the Romans, and in the 2nd century AD, Galen, physician to Marcus Aurelius, wrote on many branches of medicine and expounded the benefits of massage. He also invented cold cream by adding water to an ointment, which cooled the skin as the water evaporated (see page 79).

AROMATIC SUBSTANCES have long been burned to perfume the air and the word perfume derives from the Latin per "through" fumus "smoke". These antique incense burners are from Persia, Syria, Egypt and Turkey.

FRAGRANCES OF ASIA

Aromatic oils have been used in Chinese herbalism for thousands of years – the Great Herbal from around 200BC, which is named after the legendary Shen Nong, lists 365 plants used medicinally.

Throughout Asia, perfumes have always been prized for their medicinal and cosmetic properties: a still found in the Himalayan foothills indicates that the distillation of essential oils prospered in 3000BC, and in modern bazaars from Istanbul to Bombay, oils and aromatic remedies are abundant. In the 9th century, Baghdad, in modern-day Iraq, was the centre of the rose industry, and thrived on the export of rose water to India. Avicenna, a philosopher and physician born in AD980 in Bukhara, in modern-day Uzbekistan, is credited with improving the rose distillation process through his invention of the refrigerated coil. He also wrote numerous books on health, including the *Kitab al-Qanun*, or Canon of Medicine, in which the action of medicinal and aromatic plants and spices was explored.

India has a long tradition of using aromatic plants, and the holistic system of Ayurvedic medicine, which views health as a balance between person and environment, often combines scented oils and spices with massage.

ESSENTIAL OILS IN EUROPE

By the 12th century, with the influence of the Crusades, trade routes had developed with the Middle East, bringing an influx of spices, herbs and exotic scents. Herb gardens were cultivated in monasteries, and monks and nuns prepared popular remedies such as Carmelite water made with melissa. From the Middle Ages on, numerous herbals, categorizing plants and their therapeutic remedies, were compiled, including those of herbalists Nicholas Culpeper (1652), William Turner (1568) and John Gerard (1597).

In the 18th century, aromatic vinegars and perfumed waters gained in popularity, especially Eau de Cologne, a favourite of Napoleon and considered an elixir of life. Four grave-robbers from Marseilles had earlier

THIS ENGRAVING from 1898 shows the commercial production of rose oil, which began in Grasse in the south of France in the 18th century.

won notoriety for a vinegar recipe which they claimed protected them from the plague (see page 84).

In the early 20th century, Réné Gattefossé, a French chemist working in his family perfumery, became fascinated by the therapeutic properties of essential oils when, after burning his hands, he rinsed them with lavender essence, which stopped "the gasification of the tissues". He studied the antiseptic, bactericidal, anti-viral and anti-inflammatory properties of essential oils, and in 1937 introduced the term *aromatherapie*.

During World Wars I and II, essential oils were used to treat wounds, and in the 1960s, Dr. Jean Valnet, one of the French doctors who pioneered this work, published his findings on essential oils. Austrian biochemist Marguerite Maury studied Valnet's work and introduced aromatherapy to Britain. She continued research into the benefits of essential oils for health and beauty, created the concept of the individual prescription (see page 15), and re-kindled the ancient link between aromatherapy and massage.

HARVESTING & EXTRACTION

Essential oils, occasionally referred to as essences, volatile oils or ethereal oils, are extracted from aromatic plants which are commercially cultivated throughout the world. Turkey and Bulgaria are famous for rose oil, India for jasmine, and the island of Réunion for geranium, while tea tree oil is associated with Australia, and mint with the U.S.A. However, the essential oil industry is especially vulnerable to vagaries of climate and, like any industry, to political upheaval, and the sources of specific oils have changed many times through history.

CLIMATE & HARVESTING

The production of essential oils can be variable, but on average, 70 kg (154 lb) of plant material produces around 2 litres (3½ pints) of essential oil. As plants are at the mercy of weather and soil conditions, their yield and quality varies from year to year. In 1970, for instance, the geranium crop of Réunion was ruined by a cyclone. Réunion's inability to supply the oil led to a shortage, causing the price to increase, which in turn prompted other countries, such as Egypt, to cultivate geraniums. The yield of essential oil also depends on the time of harvesting. Certain plants, such as ylang ylang, are picked early in the morning when they are most aromatic. Others, including jasmine, are harvested at night, when their scent is strongest. Some plants, such as rose, are processed at source so as not to lose any volatile oils, while others, such as juniper, must first be dried and may be exported for distillation.

EXTRACTION

Steam distillation is the most common method of extraction. Plant material is heated by steam in a still, and the volatile parts present in the plant evaporate into the steam. These vapours are carried along a closed outlet, and are cooled and condensed by being passed through a cold water jacket. The resulting water is collected in a flask and the essential oil floats on the surface. Flower water is a by-product.
In solvent extraction, plant material is placed in a drum with a hydrocarbon solvent to dissolve the essential oil. The solution is filtered off and concentrated by distillation, leaving behind either a "concrete", a combination of wax and essential oil, or a "resinoid", a substance containing resin. A second

process of solvent extraction using pure alcohol recovers most of the oil. The alcohol is then evaporated, leaving a solution called "absolute".

The phytonic process is a new, highly efficient and economical form of solvent extraction developed in Britain by Dr. Peter Wilde. Environmentally friendly solvents are used at room temperature in a sealed apparatus to extract essential oil, "phytol", from plants.

Super-critical carbon dioxide extraction uses carbon dioxide gas at very high pressure to dissolve essential oil from a wide range of plant material. This supersedes the liquid form of the chemical developed in the 1970s. The equipment is massive and extremely expensive, but there are several process plants around the world producing oils of excellent quality.

Expression is a process used to extract essential oil from citrus fruits. The rind of the fruit is crushed to release the essential oil just under the surface.

Enfleurage, now nearly obsolete, involved pressing flowers into fat-coated glass plates. The flowers were replaced daily until the fat was saturated with essential oil, which was then dissolved from the fat with alcohol.

TODAY, LAVENDER FIELDS are usually harvested by slow-moving machines. They begin picking the flowers early in the morning and continue throughout the day. Roughly 200 kg (440 lb) of lavender flowers are needed to produce about six litres (10½ pints) of essential oil, using the process of steam distillation.

A TRADITIONAL PROCESS of extraction, known as maceration and filtration, is employed at the Fragonard perfumery in Grasse, France. Plant material is placed in hot oil, which absorbs the plant's aromatic essence. The plant material is removed and the process is repeated until the oil is perfumed.

CARRIER OILS & BLENDING

Carrier oils are used to dilute essential oils for use in aromatherapy massage and to make beauty preparations. Containing vitamins, proteins and minerals, they are highly effective moisturizers and provide many of the nutrients that the skin needs to keep it smooth and supple. Cold-pressed carrier oils are usually of a higher quality than heat- or solvent-extracted oils.

ALL-PURPOSE CARRIER OILS

These viscous carrier oils can be used alone, or enriched with special oils to dilute essential oils for use in aromatherapy massage, cosmetics or in a fragrant bath.

Apricot kernel oil, extracted from the apricot kernel, is rich in minerals and vitamins. A natural moisturizer, it has a light texture and high penetrative qualities.
Sunflower oil is a lovely fine oil which I use in most of my blends for body massage. It contains vitamin E.
Soya oil, extracted from the soya bean plant, is light, nourishing and easily absorbed. It is especially suited to oily skin.
Sweet almond oil is extracted from the almond kernel and has soothing, softening properties. Always use the sweet, not bitter, variety. It has been popular throughout history and is suitable for babies.
Grapeseed oil, extracted from the seeds of muscat raisins by heat, is good for oily skin.

SPECIAL CARRIER OILS

These special oils can be added to the all-purpose oils to improve penetration of the skin, nourish dry, dehydrated skin, or extend the life of an oil blend.

Carrot oil is rich in vitamins, especially A. Add only 10% to other carrier oils, otherwise its bright orange colour can temporarily stain the skin.
Sesame oil, extracted from the raw sesame seed, has a slightly nutty aroma and contains 85% unsaturated and 15% saturated fatty acids. It can be added to other oils to enrich them. Do not use the heavy-scented brown oil from the cooked seed.
Avocado oil is extracted from the flesh of the avocado. It is rich in vitamins A and B, and in lecithin, proteins and fatty acids. An excellent skin softener, it is easily absorbed.

Jojoba is a natural liquid wax from the kernels of an evergreen desert plant and it has a chemical composition resembling the skin's sebum. Its waxy structure and anti-bacterial properties give it a long shelf-life. Readily absorbed by the skin, it has a non-greasy softening effect and is especially suitable for the face. It is also good for thickening creams.
Wheatgerm oil is rich and viscous, but its rather strong smell can be difficult to mask. Add 10-20% of wheatgerm oil to other carrier oils to guard against rancidity and prolong the life of a blend.

Sunflower oil

Sweet almond oil

Sesame oil

Jojoba

Apricot kernel oil

Soya oil

Grapeseed oil

Carrot oil

Avocado oil

Wheatgerm oil

CHOOSING ESSENTIAL OILS

An oil blend is made by mixing a few drops of essential oil with one of the carrier oils opposite. We all like different scents, and it is essential that the aroma of the blend appeals to you, or to your friend if you are blending oils before giving a massage. Create what Marguerite Maury (see page 11) called an individual prescription. First decide what effect you are hoping to achieve: do you want the aroma to sedate or revive, to energize or to calm? Do you want to use oils for their therapeutic properties or simply to pamper? Then,

referring to pages 17–39, make a list of essential oils suited to your requirements. Select two or three from your list – good blends usually combine all three notes: top (gives the initial scent), middle (rounds out the blend) and base (released last, this acts as a fixative). The general rule is that little is best: a weak blend of oils often smells better, and is therefore more effective, than a stronger blend. Follow the guide below to achieve the safest dilution of essential oils for a balanced fragrance and maximum therapeutic benefit.

BLENDING OILS

Oil blends are usually divided into normal and low dilutions. Aromatherapists refer to these dilutions as percentages, based on the amount of essential oil in carrier oil, and there is a simple way to work them out. To calculate how many drops of essential oil are needed to make a normal dilution of 2½%, divide the number of millilitres of carrier oil by 2; for a low dilution of 1%, divide by 4. Most essential oil bottles come with a dropper for easy measuring. Refer to the individual essential oil entries on pages 18–39, paying special attention to the cautions listed, for special instructions on which dilution to use. For a full body massage, 20ml of oil is needed; for the face, 10 ml is enough. You can make larger quantities and store them (see overleaf).

MAKING AN OIL BLEND

1 Choose a carrier oil (or blend of carrier oils) based on your skin type and determine the amount you will need. Decant the carrier oil into a dark bottle a little larger than the amount of oil.

2 Choose 2–3 essential oils based on the effect you require, and calculate the number of drops to use. Add to the carrier oil. Close the bottle and label it clearly. Shake well before use.

BLENDING GUIDE

Normal dilution of 2½%:

ml carrier oil ÷ 2 = total drops essential oil
(e.g. 20 ml carrier oil ÷ 2 = 10 drops essential oil)

SAMPLE 2½% BLEND

Essential Oils
5 drops sandalwood
3 drops lavender
2 drops orange
Carrier Oil
20 ml apricot kernel

TOTAL: 10 drops essential oil per 20 ml carrier oil

Low dilution of 1% for sensitive skin and for use during pregnancy:

ml carrier oil ÷ 4 = total drops essential oil
(e.g. 20 ml carrier oil ÷ 4 = 5 drops essential oil)

SAMPLE 1% BLEND

Essential Oils
3 drops rosemary
1 drop each of lemon-grass and juniper
Carrier Oil
20 ml sunflower oil

TOTAL: 5 drops essential oil per 20 ml carrier oil

Extremely low dilution for very sensitive skin, children & babies:

Use just 1 drop essential oil per 10 ml carrier oil, or use sweet almond oil by itself.

STORAGE & SAFETY

It is a common misconception that anything natural is safe. Yet many dangerous poisons are natural, and almost anything used in excess can be harmful. Since essential oils are highly concentrated, they need to be used with care. Before you start to use essential oils, read these guidelines to ensure that your oil blends and treatments will be successful and enjoyable.

STORAGE

Essential oils are highly volatile and evaporate easily. As heat, air and light affect them, they should be kept in dark glass bottles in normal to cool temperatures (65°F/18°C). Although some wood oils can improve with age, most oils slowly deteriorate and should be used within a couple of years. They can be stored in the bottom of the refrigerator to prolong their life. Do not worry if they solidify – they will liquefy at room temperature. Citrus oils should be used within a year. Once the essential oils have been diluted in a carrier oil, their shelf-life is reduced to a few months.

LABEL all oil blends

STORAGE GUIDELINES

- Store oils in dark glass bottles in a cool, dark place with the lids tightly secured to prevent evaporation
- Label bottles with the oils, dilution and date
- Store out of the reach of children
- Essential oils are flammable, so keep them away from naked flames
- Do not store on polished surfaces, as the oils can leave marks; wipe up spills immediately.

PATCH TEST

Place a drop of diluted essential oil (2½%) on the inside of your wrist or the crease of your elbow. Cover with a sticking plaster and examine after 12 hours. If there is any redness or itching, do not use the oil. If you have an adverse reaction to an oil, apply almond oil to the area, then wash with cold water.

SAFETY

Essential oils should always be diluted. It is possible to irritate the skin by using too strong a concentration of oil. To avoid possible irritation or allergic reaction, carry out a patch test (see below, left) before using a new essential oil on yourself or a friend, and adhere strictly to the recommended dilutions (see page 15).

SAFETY PRECAUTIONS

- Keep essential oils away from children and pets
- Never take essential oils internally unless prescribed by a medically qualified aromatherapist
- Do not apply oils to the skin neat. The only exception is spot application of one drop of lavender or tea tree oil with a cotton wool bud on stings, spots or cuts
- Do not rub your eyes after using essential oils; if oil gets in the eye, rinse at once with cool water
- During pregnancy, consult a doctor and qualified aromatherapist as some oils should be avoided; use low dilutions (1% or less) of gentle oils such as chamomile, citrus oils, frankincense, geranium, lavender, sandalwood and rose
- If you suffer from epilepsy, consult a doctor before using essential oils; check the cautions for each oil before use, as some are stimulants
- Use the recommended mild oils (see pages 19, 20 and 31) for young children in extremely low dilutions (1% or less) and consult a qualified aromatherapist
- For sensitive skin, use well-diluted oils (1%)
- Citrus oils increase sensitivity to the sun, so avoid sun and sunbeds for six hours after use
- If taking homeopathic medicine, consult a homeopath before using essential oils; oils may reduce effectiveness
- Avoid prolonged use of the same essential oil.

A CATALOGUE OF OILS

An illustrated catalogue of over 20 of my favourite essential oils follows, arranged in alphabetical order by the botanical names of the plants from which the oils are extracted. The catalogue includes photographs of the plant source and essential oil, with details of the note, expense, scent and chemical constituents. There are historical anecdotes and the latest scientific research, as well as details of the principal therapeutic uses, a suitable massage and compatible essential oils to use in blends. Key information is listed and explained below.

USING THE CATALOGUE

① BOTANICAL NAME
Sometimes more than one name appears, as certain essential oils have more than one plant source.

② THERAPEUTIC PROPERTIES
This is a guide to traditional uses of essential oils and modern scientific research. It is divided into sections that explain how the oils are used, with cross-references to more practical sections of the book.

③ OIL COMBINATIONS
Three complementary oils are suggested for use in an oil blend to enhance the essential oil featured.

④ SCENT
This describes the fragrance of the essential oil.

⑤ NOTES
In *The Art of Perfumery* (1862), Septimus Piesse classified scents as musical notes. In this now-simplified system, top notes are the first impressions of a scent, middle notes are the body, and base notes are lasting fragrances. One oil can represent all three notes; the colour bar varies from weak to strong to reflect the intensity of the notes.

⑥ EXPENSE RATING
One star indicates the least expensive oil, and four stars the most expensive. The price reflects the yield of oil in the plant, but it does not guarantee quality. Trust your sense of smell and the integrity of your supplier.

⑦ CAUTIONS
Any cautions unique to a particular oil are stated here, but before using any essential oil, read the safety guidelines on page 16.

⑧ PLANT SOURCE
The plant from which the oil is extracted is shown, with details of which part is used and how the oil is extracted.

⑨ COLOUR RANGE
Essential oils vary from clear to dark blue to bright orange.

⑩ MAIN CONSTITUENTS
Essential oils have a complex chemical make-up, and not all elements have been identified. The main constituents include terpenes and their derivatives (alcohols, esters, aldehydes, ketones, phenols). These feature widely in essential oils. Oils with high levels of alcohols and esters, such as clary sage, have gentle, healing properties. Aldehydes, ketones and phenols are therapeutically active, but oils with these constituents, such as lemongrass, should be used in low concentrations.
Of the other constituents, monoterpenes, including camphene and limonene, have anti-viral properties, while sesquiterpenes are less volatile and have a stronger odour.

⑪ SUITABLE MASSAGE
A massage is suggested for a part of the body where the oil is especially effective.

FRANKINCENSE

Boswellia carterii / Boswellia thurifera

The earliest record of frankincense is a relief in a magnificent temple in Upper Egypt, built in the 15th century BC by Queen Hatshepsut. The relief illustrates an expedition to Punt, on the coast of modern-day Somalia, to collect the precious gum. Frankincense was used extensively in temple rituals, and as a perfume and medicine. It is a key element of incense and plays a part in holy rituals today.

SCENT
Balsamic, rich, sweet, warm

NOTE		
BASE	MIDDLE	TOP

EXPENSE RATING
✳ ✳

CAUTIONS
See page 16.

Main constituents:
monoterpenes, olibanol, pinene, camphene, limonene, resinous substances

THERAPEUTIC PROPERTIES

Frankincense, called olibanum in the Arabian Peninsula and Ethiopia where it originates, is noted for remarkable healing effects on the skin and respiratory tract. Chinese healers used it to treat infected sores and leprosy.

In 1981 some German scientists investigated the "mind bending" effects of inhaling the aroma, and found that a psychoactive substance is produced when the gum is burned. Frankincense also deepens breathing, which can result in calmness, and this could explain how using it as incense creates a state conducive to prayer.

EMOTIONS & MIND

I'll never forget my excitement when, walking in northern Kenya, I came across a frankincense tree and was able to pick off some of the pale yellow resin. Its rich, rejuvenating fragrance helped me to complete that day's hike.

ACHES & PAINS

In India, frankincense has been, and still is, used to treat rheumatism.

RESPIRATORY PROBLEMS

Anti-inflammatory, antiseptic and anti-fungal. The oil causes the bronchii of the lungs to dilate, and may relieve the discomfort of lung infections. Once inhaled, it acts upon mucus, enabling sputum to be expelled from the body. Use diluted oil in a chest massage.

SKIN & BEAUTY

Traditionally, frankincense has been used as a perfume base. An Asian friend perfumes her damp hair with the fragrance of the burnt oil. I add

Boswellia carterii

DROPLETS OF GUM RESIN form when the bark of the frankincense tree is scraped. They harden and solidify, then oil is obtained from the resin.

the oil to face products for its lovely perfume and because it is thought to have rejuvenating properties. Add it to a massage oil or cream for dry or ageing skin (see page 80).

CHEST MASSAGE

A chest massage with frankincense can deepen breathing (see pages 58–59).

OIL COMBINATIONS

Sandalwood   Geranium   Rose

SANDALWOOD OIL enhances the woody, resinous scent of frankincense oil, while geranium and rose oils sweeten the aroma.

Chamaemelum nobile / Matricaria recutita
CHAMOMILE

O ne of the gentlest of oils, chamomile has a very soothing effect and is well suited to treating children. It was revered by the Ancient Egyptians and has long been associated with herbal medicine. According to the herbalist Nicholas Culpeper, writing in The English Physician *(1652), "bathing with a decoction of chamomile taketh away weariness and easeth pain".*

SCENT
Pungent, herbaceous, fruity

NOTE
MIDDLE

EXPENSE RATING
✳ ✳ ✳

CAUTIONS
See page 16.

Main constituents:
chamazulene, bisabolol, esters, pinene, linalol

THERAPEUTIC PROPERTIES

This oil is my first choice when needing to calm and soothe. Roman chamomile (*Chamaemelum nobile*) has a high ester content, making it especially soothing. The deep blue colour of the oil of German chamomile (*Matricaria recutita*) comes from its high level of chamazulene, which boosts its anti-inflammatory effect. Chamomile is grown in temperate parts of Europe and Eurasia, Egypt and the U.S.A.

Matricaria recutita

——— EMOTIONS & MIND ———
Use in massage blends to ease anxiety, insomnia, and stress-related headaches and pre-menstrual tension.

——— ACHES & PAINS ———
Soothes muscular aches, sprains and swollen joints (see pages 100–1).

——— DIGESTIVE PROBLEMS ———
Anti-spasmodic. Use to treat colic, flatulence and indigestion. Massage the abdomen gently with diluted oil.

——— SKIN & BEAUTY ———
Suitable for all skin types. Antiseptic; has healing properties when applied diluted to inflamed or grazed skin. Excellent remedy for acne, eczema, psoriasis (see pages 108–9), and for allergies, rashes and chapped nipples.

FACIAL MASSAGE

Soothing chamomile oil enhances facial treatments (see pages 74–83).

OIL COMBINATIONS

Geranium

Clary sage

Lavender

CHAMOMILE OIL has a powerful aroma, so very little is needed. Geranium, clary sage and lavender all soften the aroma, while clary sage and lavender also reinforce its sedative nature.

Chamaemelum nobile

THE FLOWERS *of both varieties of chamomile are distilled to extract the oil.*

Citrus aurantium / Citrus bigaradia / Citrus vulgaris

ORANGE, NEROLI & PETITGRAIN

Native to Asia, the bitter, or Seville, orange tree is thought to have been introduced to Europe along Arab trade routes around AD1200. The tree gained popularity in Spain under Moorish rule, but as oranges were scarce and expensive, they were not greatly used in European herbal medicine until the late 17th century. By the 18th century, they were being recommended for an enormous variety of complaints, ranging from melancholia to heart problems and colic. The tree yields three essential citrus oils: orange, neroli, and petitgrain. Today all are used to calm the nerves and combat insomnia.

Citrus aurantium, Citrus bigaradia, Citrus vulgaris

ORANGE

THERAPEUTIC PROPERTIES
Historically, this citrus oil was used in Europe as a mild tonic to treat the nerves, bronchitis and digestive problems, as it still is in traditional Chinese medicine.

—— **EMOTIONS & MIND** ——
Orange is considered a general tonic. The uplifting, familiar scent can allay anxiety and is popular with children.

—— **DIGESTIVE PROBLEMS** ——
Its anti-spasmodic action helps to reduce colic and heartburn. To treat constipation and indigestion, massage the abdomen with diluted oil.

Citrus aurantium

ORANGE OIL is expressed from the rind of the bitter orange fruit.

—— **SKIN & BEAUTY** ——
Mildly astringent. Use orange oil in facial creams or oils for facial massage to bring vitality to the skin.

Main constituents: limonene, myrcene, citral, citronellal

SCENT
Fresh, citrus-like, dry

NOTE
BASE   MIDDLE   TOP

EXPENSE RATING
*

CAUTIONS
Avoid sun / sunbeds for 6 hours; can cause allergies. See page 16.

BACK MASSAGE

Orange oil, like neroli and petitgrain, can ease stress in the back (see pages 48–53).

OIL COMBINATIONS

Juniper

Frankincense

Cypress

FRANKINCENSE AND JUNIPER add spice to orange oil, and cypress provides a clean, fresh scent.

Citrus aurantium, Citrus bigaradia

NEROLI

THERAPEUTIC PROPERTIES

One of the most exquisite scents, neroli is prized for its gentle sedative nature. The oil is said to be named after the wife of the Italian prince of Nerola, who used it extensively.

EMOTIONS & MIND

Extremely beneficial in treating panic attacks and insomnia (see pages 98–99).

DIGESTIVE PROBLEMS

For stress-related disturbances, such as irritable bowel syndrome, gently massage the abdomen with diluted oil.

SKIN & BEAUTY

Valuable in skin-care preparations, particularly for mature or sensitive skin and for broken capillaries.

NEROLI OIL *is distilled from the blossom of the bitter orange tree.*

Citrus aurantium

OIL COMBINATIONS

Benzoin

Lavender

Frankincense

BENZOIN AND FRANKINCENSE deepen the scent of neroli, and lavender enhances its sedative qualities.

Main constituents: *linalol, limonene, linalyl acetate, nerol, geraniol*

SCENT
Intensely sweet, rich, floral

NOTE		
BASE	MIDDLE	TOP

EXPENSE RATING
✳ ✳ ✳ ✳

CAUTIONS
See page 16.

Citrus aurantium

PETITGRAIN

THERAPEUTIC PROPERTIES

Petitgrain oil resembles neroli therapeutically and is also good for nervous and stress-related conditions, including insomnia, and jet lag. Both are frequently used in high-quality Eau de Cologne. Being cheaper and less intense in aroma than neroli, it is also popular in massage oils.

EMOTIONS & MIND

I use petitgrain for its ability to relieve stress. It is lovely in a bath oil to banish fatigue and relieve anxiety.

SKIN & BEAUTY

Especially good for irritated skin and acne. Use it in a facial massage or add to home-made face creams (see page 72). It also makes a good hair tonic — add 12 drops to the final rinse.

PETITGRAIN OIL *is distilled from the leaves and green twigs of the bitter orange tree.*

OIL COMBINATIONS

Rosemary   **Clary sage**

Geranium

GERANIUM OIL rounds out the aroma of petitgrain, while rosemary oil adds sharpness, and clary sage enhances its sedative effects.

Main constituents: *linalyl acetate, linalol, limonene, geraniol, terpineol*

SCENT
Floral, citrus-like, woody

NOTE		
BASE	MIDDLE	TOP

EXPENSE RATING
✳

CAUTIONS
See page 16.

Citrus bergamia
BERGAMOT

*W*idely used in Italian folk medicine, bergamot takes its name from an Italian village where it was used traditionally for reducing fevers. The delightful perfume is an important ingredient in Eau de Cologne and the citrus oil is used to flavour Earl Grey tea. Bergamot oil has an uplifting effect that seems to help allay depression, and nearly everyone likes its fresh, citrus-like aroma.

SCENT
Fresh, lively, citrus-like

NOTE
BASE   MIDDLE   **TOP**

EXPENSE RATING
✳ ✳

CAUTIONS
Use low dilutions (1%); avoid sun & sunbeds for 6 hours. See page 16.

Main constituents: linalyl acetate, limonene, linalol, bergaptene

THERAPEUTIC PROPERTIES

The oil from bergamot, which is cultivated in Italy, South America and west Africa, lifts the spirits and helps to heal wounds and skin problems. Through his research in the 1960s and 70s, the Italian doctor, Paolo Rosvesti, confirmed that it helps to relieve depressive states and anxiety. Indian research found that bergamot also helps to regulate the appetite.

Its delightful scent makes bergamot popular as an air freshener, with the added benefit that its antiseptic and anti-viral properties may protect against airborne bacteria. I burn the oil in a vaporizer in the classroom to help new students feel at ease.

Bergaptene, one of the constituents of the oil, can cause photosensitivity, so wait at least six hours after use before exposing yourself to the sun or a sunbed (and preferably wash first). A bergaptene-free oil is also available.

EMOTIONS & MIND
Noted for its excellent calming and anti-depressant qualities, which are due to a high ester content. Like most citrus oils, bergamot helps to improve moods and lift depression. Seems to allay anxiety and grief, especially when used in conjunction with a relaxing face or back massage.

URINARY PROBLEMS
Antiseptic. Add well-diluted oil (1%) to the bath to treat cystitis.

SKIN & BEAUTY
Its antiseptic properties make bergamot useful in the treatment of acne. Gently stroke the face to

THE OIL is expressed from the peel of the fruit when nearly ripe, but still green.

stimulate the circulation and lymphatic flow. Bergamot oil's delightful, fresh scent may help to alleviate the stress suffered by those with skin problems. The famous French herbalist, Maurice Mességué, writing in 1975 recommended it as an excellent disinfectant for wounds, abscesses and boils (see pages 102–3). The essential oil may cause skin irritation so use it in low dilutions of 1% or less; never apply it neat.

OIL COMBINATIONS

Juniper

Neroli

Chamomile

BERGAMOT OIL blends with juniper to reinforce its use as an air purifier. Chamomile oil enhances its calming effect, and neroli oil adds depth to the refreshing citrus-like perfume.

FACIAL MASSAGE

The uplifting effect of bergamot oil enhances facials (see pages 74–79).

Cupressus sempervirens
CYPRESS

*I*n many cultures, the cypress tree has represented eternal life, and Plato (c.429–347BC) referred to it as the symbol of immortality. The oil has a fresh, spicy aroma that many people find refreshing, and in Ancient Greece it was customary to send tuberculosis patients into a cypress grove to breathe the air and ease their symptoms. Cypress oil is still used to treat respiratory complaints.

SCENT
Spicy, sweet, balsamic, refreshing

NOTE
BASE   MIDDLE   **TOP**

EXPENSE RATING
*

CAUTIONS
Avoid in the first three months of pregnancy. See page 16.

Main constituents: pinene, carene, myrcene, camphene, sylvestrene

THERAPEUTIC PROPERTIES

Cypress was burned as incense in the ancient world for purification, and was used because of its anti-spasmodic properties to treat respiratory problems. In traditional Chinese and Indian Ayurvedic medicine, it was recognized for its astringent effects.

In 1597 John Gerard, herbalist to King James I of England, wrote in *The Herball or Generall Historie of Plantes* that "the leaves and nuts are good to cure the rupture" and today the oil is used to treat haemorrhoids, varicose veins, broken capillaries and bruising. Since the 16th century, cypress has been advocated as an insect repellent. Gerard also advised people to "use the smoke of the leaves to drive away gnats… and the wood laid amongst garments preserveth against the moths".

—ACHES & PAINS —
I have found it useful in massage blends to treat rheumatic aches; or in a cold compress when massage is inadvisable, for example in reducing the spread of recent bruising, on varicose veins, or when rheumatic joints are inflamed.

FOOT MASSAGE

Cypress oil helps to inhibit sweat and revitalize tired feet (see pages 66–67).

OIL COMBINATIONS

Citrus oils   *Rose*   *Frankincense*

CYPRESS OIL blends well with all citrus oils in tonics and with rose oil for facial massage blends, while frankincense brings out the incense-like nature of the aroma.

THE NEEDLES and twigs of the tree are distilled to extract the oil.

— RESPIRATORY PROBLEMS —
Anti-spasmodic. Eases coughs, asthma, bronchitis and sore throats. Put a couple of drops on a handkerchief and inhale deeply.

SKIN & BEAUTY
Astringent; good for oily skin. I find the aroma of cypress oil appeals particularly to men. Use in facial steaming, skin tonics or aftershaves. Often included in anti-cellulite blends (see pages 106–7). Helpful for people who suffer from sweaty feet. Add a couple of drops to a daily foot bath, or massage the feet with diluted oil.

Cymbopogon citratus
LEMON-GRASS

A traditional ingredient in Malaysian and Thai cooking, lemon-grass is also the source of an essential oil that has valuable therapeutic uses. In addition to acting as a digestive tonic, diuretic and antiseptic, the oil has pain-relieving properties. Combined with massage, the powerful lemony aroma makes a great restorative for physical and emotional problems. Men especially like its strong, fresh scent.

SCENT
Lemony, grassy, dry, fresh

NOTE

BASE	MIDDLE	TOP

EXPENSE RATING
*

CAUTIONS
Possible skin irritation, use low dilutions (1%). See page 16.

Main constituents: citral, linalol, geraniol, myrcene, citronellal

THERAPEUTIC PROPERTIES

Lemon-grass is considered a cooling herb in India and citral, its major constituent, has sedative and antiseptic effects. In India, it is used widely in Ayurvedic medicine to treat fevers and infections, and recent research here has confirmed the oil's analgesic and antifungal properties and its ability to reduce fevers. Use with caution on the face, neck and delicate skin. Lemon-grass is cultivated in Africa, Asia and the West Indies.

EMOTIONS & MIND
Acts as a sedative on the central nervous system. Use to counteract mental fatigue (see pages 98–99).

ACHES & PAINS
I use well-diluted lemon-grass oil to massage athletes after sport, especially if they are drained of energy.

DIGESTIVE PROBLEMS
Considered to be a tonic for the digestive system. Massage a well-diluted oil blend into the abdomen.

SKIN & BEAUTY
Antiseptic. Lemon-grass oil is used for treating acne (see pages 108–9).

ABDOMEN MASSAGE

Use lemon-grass in a massage oil blend as a tonic for the digestion (see page 88).

OIL COMBINATIONS

Sandalwood

Rose

Rosemary

LEMON-GRASS OIL blends well with rose and sandalwood oils, which soften its strong aroma, and with rosemary oil, which enhances its refreshing scent.

LEMON-GRASS essential oil is extracted from the grass by the process of steam distillation.

Eucalyptus globulus
EUCALYPTUS

*E*asily recognized by its camphor-like vapour, eucalyptus is the classic remedy for respiratory problems and is contained in many commercial products for colds and sinus congestion. It is also used for chest complaints, musculo-skeletal problems, and to purify the air. Originally from Australia, the tree was introduced to Europe in the late 18th century, and distilled commercially in the 1850s.

SCENT
Camphor-like, sweet, woody

NOTE

BASE	MIDDLE	TOP

EXPENSE RATING
*

CAUTIONS
Use low dilutions (1%); avoid with homeopathic remedies. See page 16.

Main constituents: cineol, pinene, limonene

THERAPEUTIC PROPERTIES

Traditionally, Australian Aboriginal peoples bound the leaves of the indigenous eucalyptus tree to wounds to speed healing. Recent research has confirmed the oil's pain-relieving and anti-inflammatory properties, and its ability to reduce swelling and accelerate healing.

ACHES & PAINS

Eucalyptus oil feels cool to the skin, but warm to the muscles (see pages 100–1). The cineol content makes it analgesic, and the oil also reduces fevers.

RESPIRATORY PROBLEMS

The main constituent of eucalyptus essential oil, cineol, is responsible for its powerful antiseptic, anti-viral and expectorant effects. Use in a steam inhalation (see pages 102–3), put two drops on a handkerchief and inhale, or massage the chest with diluted oil.

ALLERGIES & INFECTIONS

It has anti-bacterial properties, is a good anti-viral agent and stimulates the immune system. When used in a vaporizer, the essential oil reduces airborne microbes.

OIL COMBINATIONS

Marjoram

Lavender

Juniper

MARJORAM OIL boosts the decongestant effect of eucalyptus oil, juniper oil adds a clean scent, and lavender softens the aroma and enhances the harmony of the blend.

CHEST MASSAGE

The powerful scent relaxes the chest and can ease congestion (see pages 58–59).

THE LEAVES of the plant, cultivated in Australia and southern Europe, are distilled to extract the oil.

Jasminum officinale / Jasminum grandiflorum
JASMINE

*E*xquisitely fragranced, jasmine is reputed to be an aphrodisiac. In the 16th century, the Grand Duke of Tuscany procured a plant from India. Determined to keep it to himself, he forbade his gardener to give cuttings away. Yet the gardener gave his beloved a posy containing jasmine. Delighted by its aroma, she planted the jasmine, sold cuttings and saved enough money to wed the poor gardener.

SCENT
Sweet, heady, rich, floral

NOTE
BASE	MIDDLE	TOP

EXPENSE RATING
✴ ✴ ✴ ✴

CAUTIONS
Avoid in pregnancy and on babies. Can cause headaches. See page 16.

Main constituents: benzyl acetate, linalol, linalyl acetate, jasmone

THERAPEUTIC PROPERTIES
The flowers of the jasmine plant, which is cultivated in India and North Africa, yield tiny amounts of oil, making it very expensive. It is valued in the Far East and the Indian subcontinent for its medicinal properties and scent. In China, the flowers have been used to treat dysentery and hepatitis. In Indian Ayurvedic medicine, jasmine is recommended for cleansing the blood.

Garlands of jasmine are presented to honoured guests in India and in some areas, ten days before marriage, brides are massaged daily with *Ubtan*, a blend of herbs, spices, jasmine and sweet almond oil, leaving the skin cleansed, smooth and scented with the heady aroma of jasmine.

EMOTIONS & MIND
Uplifting and stimulating. I believe the heavenly aroma acts as an anti-depressant. Use to treat lethargy (see pages 98–99).

GYNAECOLOGICAL PROBLEMS
In India, the flowers are traditionally applied to the breasts to suppress excess lactation after childbirth. For painful periods, massage the lower back and abdomen with diluted oil.

Jasminum officinale

THE STAR-SHAPED *flowers are picked at night, and oil is extracted using solvent.*

SKIN & BEAUTY
Jasmine oil is frequently used in skin-care preparations for its delicious perfume and invigorating effect (see page 75).

SCALP MASSAGE

Use jasmine oil in a refreshing massage to perfume the scalp (see page 85).

OIL COMBINATIONS

Clary sage   *Sandalwood*   *Citrus oils*

CLARY SAGE emphasizes the sensual aspect of the oil. In India, jasmine oil is traditionally blended with exotic sandalwood oil, while citrus oils freshen its aroma.

Juniperus communis

JUNIPER

*R*enowned *for its cleansing properties, juniper has been used through the ages to purify body, mind and spirit. It has been valued by all the great civilizations since Ancient Egyptian times to fight infection and for purification ceremonies (sprigs with berries were said to keep witches away). Its anti-viral properties make juniper useful in treating respiratory infections and an ideal air freshener.*

SCENT
Woody, fresh, sweet

NOTE
BASE   **MIDDLE**   TOP

EXPENSE RATING
*

CAUTIONS
Avoid in pregnancy, kidney disease or glomerulonephritis. See page 16.

Main constituents: pinene, myrcene, limonene

THERAPEUTIC PROPERTIES

In Ancient Greece, juniper was burned as incense to combat epidemics, as it was in a German cholera outbreak in 1856, and a smallpox epidemic in France in 1870. Cato the Elder (234–149BC), a Roman, considered the berries to be diuretic as did Gerard, writing that "it provoketh urine". Culpeper said the plant "provokes urine exceedingly… helps the gout and sciatica, and strengthens the limbs of the body". Juniper oil is still used in similar ways.

THE BERRIES of juniper plants, cultivated in Canada and Europe, are distilled to extract the oil.

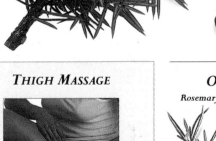

EMOTIONS & MIND

Calming and fresh. Use diluted in a bath or massage oil to ease stress.

ACHES & PAINS

Diuretic and local stimulant, useful for rheumatic problems and sports aches and pains. The constituent myrcene has analgesic properties. Dilute with a carrier oil and blend with rosemary oil for use in the bath or with ginger oil for massage (see pages 100–1).

SKIN & BEAUTY

Antiseptic; use in toners and men's aftershaves. Useful for treating acne; apply a cold compress or diluted oil. Helpful in a massage used to aid slimming or combat cellulite.

THIGH MASSAGE

Juniper oil is often used in anti-cellulite massage blends (see pages 88–89).

OIL COMBINATIONS

Rosemary

Citrus oils

Rose

ROSEMARY OIL enhances the stimulating, rubefacient effect of juniper oil, citrus oils complement its calming properties, and rose oil sweetens its scent.

Lavandula angustifolia/Lavandula officinalis
LAVENDER

Lavender is probably the most versatile and widely used essential oil. Deriving its name from the Latin lavare, *to wash, it may have been used by the Romans in bath water. Due to its sedative nature, lavender has long been recommended as a folk remedy for insomnia, for example in herbal pillows. Recently it has been employed in many hospitals to help patients relax and sleep better.*

SCENT
Sweet, floral, herbaceous, stimulating, piercing

NOTE
BASE MIDDLE TOP

EXPENSE RATING
*

CAUTIONS
See page 16.

Main constituents: linalyl acetate, linalol, caryophyllene, lavandulyl acetate, cineol, geraniol

THERAPEUTIC PROPERTIES

Lavender is used primarily for its sedative and antiseptic properties. *Lavandula officinalis* and *L. angustifolia* are known as true lavender and yield the finest oil, while *L. latifolia* and *L. fragrans* hybrids yield more oil, albeit with less sedative properties. In 1910, Réné Maurice Gattefossé, a French perfumer and chemist, rinsed his hands in lavender essence, thereby halting the onset of gangrene which had developed from a burn. His swift and successful recovery was a catalyst for research into the properties of essential oils.

THE FLOWERING tops are distilled to extract the oil.

EMOTIONS & MIND
Sedative and calming, lavender is the perfect oil to treat insomnia. Use in a massage blend, diluted in the bath, or put a drop on your pillow.

ACHES & PAINS
Analgesic, anti-spasmodic. Use in a massage blend or add diluted oil to the bath to relieve muscular aches and pains. Excellent as a headache remedy; simply massage a little oil slowly and gently around the temples.

RESPIRATORY PROBLEMS
Inhale to speed recovery from colds, bronchitis, influenza and throat infections. Use in a stimulating chest massage to relieve congestion.

SKIN & BEAUTY
Antiseptic; use to treat acne and eczema (see pages 108–9), to soothe insect bites and stings, to clean and disinfect cuts and sores, and to help heal minor burns (see pages 102–3).

OIL COMBINATIONS

Marjoram Citrus oils Frankincense

MARJORAM enhances lavender's sedative effect, citrus oils increase its floral quality, and frankincense heightens its soothing and expectorant properties.

BACK MASSAGE

A soporific massage with lavender oil can help induce sleep (see pages 48–53).

Lavandula angustifolia

Melaleuca alternifolia
TEA TREE

*T*his species of paperbark tree, native to the sub-tropical coast of New South Wales and parts of Queensland, Australia, has a long history of use as a potent antiseptic. Aboriginal peoples used poultices of the leaves on wounds and cuts, and smoked the leaves to clear congestion. Tea tree oil remains one of aromatherapy's most powerful tools in the fight against bacteria, fungi, yeast and viruses.

SCENT
Medicinal, spicy, fresh

NOTE

BASE	MIDDLE	TOP

EXPENSE RATING
*

CAUTIONS
For sensitive skin, use a normal dilution (2½%). See page 16.

Main constituents: terpineol, terpinene, cineol, cymene, pinene

THERAPEUTIC PROPERTIES

The name tea tree first appeared in Captain Cook's "Voyage towards the South Pole and around the World 1772–5". Its properties were again recognized in 1923 by Arthur Penfold, a New South Wales chemist, and several papers were published in the 1930s describing its use as a wide-spectrum antiseptic with very low toxicity. During World War II, Australian soldiers were issued with the oil, but its use declined with the advent of antibiotics after the war. From the 1970s it became popular again. Often referred to as the first-aid kit in a bottle, tea tree oil is invaluable for treating minor wounds, infections, cuts, stings and acne.

— RESPIRATORY PROBLEMS —

To relieve sore throats, coughs, sinusitis and chest congestion, place a couple of drops of tea tree oil on a handkerchief, and inhale.

— GYNAECOLOGICAL PROBLEMS —

Add diluted oil to the bath to treat cystitis, a urinary problem, and *Candida albicans*, which causes thrush.

— SKIN & BEAUTY —

For acne, dab one drop of undiluted oil on isolated spots 1–2 times a day

THE ESSENTIAL OIL is extracted from the leaves using steam distillation.

with a cotton wool bud, or use diluted in a skin tonic. For bites, stings, cuts, wounds and cold sores, apply neat oil. For athlete's foot, callouses, corns or smelly feet, add 5–10 drops to a daily foot bath. Cool minor burns with cold water, then apply neat oil.

FOOT MASSAGE

Tea tree is antiseptic and anti-fungal and so ideal for the feet (see pages 66–67).

OIL COMBINATIONS

Geranium   Lemon

Scot's pine

TEA TREE is hard to blend, but geranium sweetens its scent, Scot's pine emphasizes its spicy, medicinal aroma and lemon brings out its freshness.

Melissa officinalis
MELISSA

The delicious scent of melissa can hardly fail to lift one's spirits. I have a bush by my front door so that whenever I go in or out of the house I can take a few leaves, crush them and enjoy the effects. It is this uplifting quality of melissa, or lemon balm, that I find most therapeutic. I use it as an anti-depressant oil, especially if a client needs soothing and boosting with a general tonic.

SCENT
Soft, lemon-like, herby

NOTE
BASE   **MIDDLE**   TOP

EXPENSE RATING
✳ ✳ ✳ ✳

CAUTIONS
Possible skin irritation, so use low dilutions (1%). See page 16.

Main constituents: linalol, geraniol, citronellal, citral

THERAPEUTIC PROPERTIES

Refreshing and calming to mind and body, melissa can help those suffering from depression, anxiety, shock or bereavement. It was used in medieval "elixirs of youth" and according to Culpeper, "it causes the mind and heart to become merry…and driveth away all troublesome cares and thoughts". Cultivated in Europe and the U.S.A., the essential oil is frequently adulterated; ask your source for melissa "true" instead of melissa "type".

— EMOTIONS & MIND –
Calms, uplifts, revitalizes and restores emotional balance. Dilute well with a carrier oil and use to massage the whole body or add a few drops to bath water.

—— DIGESTIVE PROBLEMS ——
For digestive complaints that are accompanied by tension or anxiety, gently massage the abdomen with diluted melissa.

– GYNAECOLOGICAL PROBLEMS –
Thought to help regulate ovulation and menstruation, especially if irregularity is caused by emotional upset. Apply in a massage oil to the abdomen and lower back.

—— SKIN & BEAUTY ——
Antiseptic, anti-viral and anti-fungal. Relieves skin problems, including cold sores. Apply well diluted.

BACK MASSAGE

For a soothing effect, use melissa oil in a back massage (see pages 48–53).

OIL COMBINATIONS

Citrus oils

Rose

Rosemary

MELISSA combines with citrus oils to enhance its sedative qualities, and is balanced by the sharpness of rosemary and the luxurious aroma of rose.

MELISSA OIL is extracted from the leaves by steam distillation.

Mentha piperita

PEPPERMINT

*R*efreshing and energizing, peppermint reminds
me of Morocco, where it grows in abundance
and is served as a delicious tea. Peppermint is an
excellent mental stimulant, and as a digestive, it
is unsurpassed. It also helps to alleviate stomach
pains. I once used a very weak dilution of oil to
massage a baby with colic. The results were
immediate; the baby stopped crying and fell asleep.

SCENT
Minty, grass-like, balsamic, fresh

NOTE
BASE   MIDDLE   TOP

EXPENSE RATING
✳ ✳

CAUTIONS
Use low dilutions (1%); avoid with homeopathic remedies. See page 16.

Main constituents: menthol, menthone, cineol

THERAPEUTIC PROPERTIES

Research in the U.S.A. and Japan has
shown that peppermint improves
alertness and stimulates the
brain without affecting the
heart rate. This supports the
idea of Pliny the Elder (a
Roman writer born AD23) that a mint
crown could aid concentration. Mint
soothes the stomach muscles and has
long been used as a digestive. It is
cultivated in Europe and the U.S.A.

—— *EMOTIONS & MIND* ——
Improves alertness and helps
to relieve headaches. Massage
diluted oil into the temples
or add to a bath.

— *RESPIRATORY PROBLEMS* —
Powerful decongestant,
good for colds and influenza.
Massage diluted oil into
the temples or use
steam inhalation to clear
nasal passages. Prolonged
use can disturb sleep.

—— *DIGESTIVE PROBLEMS* ——
Calming, anti-spasmodic. Use
peppermint to treat flatulence,
indigestion and colic. Massage
the abdomen with low dilutions
of oil (see pages 62–63).

FOOT MASSAGE

*Use peppermint oil in a cooling massage
for tired feet (see pages 66–67).*

OIL COMBINATIONS

Rosemary

Eucalyptus

Marjoram

PEPPERMINT OIL combines perfectly with
eucalyptus and rosemary, which reinforce
its effects on colds and influenza, and with
warming and penetrating marjoram oil.

*THE LEAVES of peppermint
are partially dried before
the oil is extracted by
steam distillation.*

Origanum majorana
MARJORAM

A pungent herb from the mint family, marjoram was reputedly created by Aphrodite, the Greek goddess of love, as a symbol of happiness and well-being. If it grew on a grave, the happiness of the deceased was assured. Marjoram has been known since ancient times as a friend to the nerves and useful to women. I use the oil to calm the mind and ease taut muscles.

SCENT
Camphor-like, sweet, warm

NOTE		
BASE	MIDDLE	TOP

EXPENSE RATING
✶✶

CAUTIONS
Avoid in pregnancy; use low dilutions (1%). See page 16.

Main constituents: methyl chavicol, terpineol, eugenol, linalol and many terpenes

THERAPEUTIC PROPERTIES

Gerard and Culpeper credited marjoram with the ability to comfort and warm the brain and benefit cold, stiff joints and respiratory disorders. It is antiseptic, anti-spasmodic and anti-fungal. Japanese research has confirmed its sedative effects. Marjoram is cultivated in central and southern Europe, and Egypt.

EMOTIONS & MIND

To treat insomnia or to restore frayed nerves, use diluted oil in a warm bath or with a soothing back massage to induce a good night's sleep.

ACHES & PAINS

Wonderful for treating rheumatic aches and cold, contracted muscles, and a great antidote to aches and stiffness from over-enthusiastic exercise. Apply diluted oil in a massage, a compress, or add to the bath (see pages 100–1).

RESPIRATORY PROBLEMS

One of the best remedies to treat colds and chills. Put a few drops of oil on a handkerchief and inhale to clear sinuses and ease headaches. Use in an inhalation for bronchitis and sinusitis (see pages 102–3).

GYNAECOLOGICAL PROBLEMS

The warming and calming effects of marjoram oil help to relieve period pains. Slowly and rhythmically massage the abdomen and lower back with diluted oil or apply a warm compress to the abdomen.

LEG MASSAGE

Massage with marjoram oil eases aches (see pages 54–55, 64–65).

THE FLOWERS AND LEAVES of marjoram plants are used, and the oil is extracted by steam distillation.

OIL COMBINATIONS

Eucalyptus Lavender

Rosemary

ROSEMARY AND EUCALYPTUS OILS reinforce the benefits of marjoram to ease colds and muscular aches. Lavender enhances its sedative qualities.

Pelargonium graveolens
GERANIUM

Originating in southern Africa, geraniums were brought to Europe in the 17th century. Over 700 species exist, many of them highly perfumed. The scent of geranium oil resembles rose, with which it shares many constituents. Consequently, it is often added to rose oil to extend it. The soothing aroma helps reduce stress and, as so many people love the scent, I use it often in facial treatments.

SCENT
Sweet, round, floral, herbaceous

NOTE
BASE   MIDDLE   TOP

EXPENSE RATING
**

CAUTIONS
Use low dilutions (1%). See page 16.

Main constituents: geraniol, linalol, citronellol

THERAPEUTIC PROPERTIES

Traditionally geranium was used to staunch bleeding, heal wounds, ulcers and skin disorders and treat diarrhoea, dysentery and colic. Anti-bacterial properties and insecticidal actions were found when geranium was screened for medicinal usage in a joint project of the laboratories of the Royal Botanic Gardens, Kew and the Society of Applied Science, in Britain. I use the diluted oil for first aid on minor cuts and burns. Geranium oil is also an effective insect repellent, useful to keep in a first-aid kit.

— EMOTIONS & MIND —
Anti-depressant. It is an excellent relaxant for those suffering from nervous tension. Use the oil in inhalations, diluted in the bath or in a massage blend.

— GYNAECOLOGICAL PROBLEMS —
In a French study of 1933, it was found to be active against *Candida albicans*, which causes thrush. Can regulate mood swings associated with pre-menstrual tension (see pages 106–7).

— SKIN & BEAUTY —
Rich in the gentle alcohols, geraniol and linalol, it is suitable for all skin. Good for acne treatments due to its anti-microbial effect. Add to massage blends for the face, to skin toners and creams (see pages 70–73). Popular in anti-cellulite oils to relieve fluid retention. Gently massage the affected area.

GERANIUM OIL is extracted by steam distillation of the whole plant, cultivated in Egypt, Russia and Réunion.

OIL COMBINATIONS

Chamomile

Juniper

Citrus oils

CHAMOMILE, JUNIPER AND CITRUS OILS mellow the sweet-scented oil. Chamomile also enhances its effectiveness against cuts or inflammation.

HAND MASSAGE

The floral aroma of geranium oil leaves hands lightly fragranced (see pages 60–61).

Rosa centifolia / Rosa damascena
ROSE

*A*ccording to legend, rose oil was discovered at the wedding feast of the Mogul princess Noor Jehan. Rose water poured into a canal encircling the garden separated in the sun's heat and the bridal couple gathered the droplets of aromatic oil. Since antiquity, the healing virtues of rose oil have been celebrated, but its exquisite scent still cannot be synthetically made: it has about 300 constituents, not all known.

SCENT
Intense, lingering, rosy floral

NOTE

BASE	MIDDLE	TOP

EXPENSE RATING
✶ ✶ ✶ ✶

CAUTIONS
See page 16.

Main constituents: citronellol, geraniol, nerol, linalol, citral, eugenol, phenyl ethanol

THERAPEUTIC PROPERTIES

Roses have long been associated with Venus, Roman goddess of love and beauty, and the oil is still used in beauty products. Avicenna, the 10th-century philosopher and physician, said rose oil "increases the might of the brain and quickes the mind". As the oil yield from roses is low (0.02%), it is extremely costly. For therapeutic use, oil distilled without heat, "phytol", or by steam, "otto", is best: oil extracted by solvent, "absolute", is less pure.

EMOTIONS & MIND

Anti-depressant. A 1969 Bulgarian study found that rose oil increases alertness and gives sweeter dreams.

DIGESTIVE PROBLEMS

In Bulgaria it is used as a liver tonic; in China, as a cure for liver stagnation. Eases hangovers (see pages 104–5).

GYNAECOLOGICAL PROBLEMS

A soothing, relaxing massage with rose oil helps to ease pre-menstrual tension.

SKIN & BEAUTY

Antihistamine, antiseptic. Use in face massage and skin products to calm and uplift (see page 75). A rose water compress can ease signs of stress in the face by relieving headaches, eye strain and inflammation.

OIL COMBINATIONS

Sandalwood

Lavender

Chamomile

THE BEAUTIFUL PIERCING SCENT OF ROSE combines perfectly with lavender and chamomile, which bring out its freshness. Sandalwood makes it deeper and more exotic.

Rosa centifolia

THE FLOWERS are the source of the oil: 200 kg (440 lb) of petals produce about 1 litre (1¾ pints) of rose otto. Most roses come from Bulgaria, France, Morocco, Turkey and Russia.

FACIAL MASSAGE

Soothing rose oil has a cooling effect on the face (see pages 74–79).

Rosmarinus officinalis
ROSEMARY

*R*evered as the herb sacred to remembrance, rosemary was said by Culpeper to "help a weak memory and quicken the senses". In medieval times, it was strewn on the floor and carried in posies to inhale in oppressive conditions. The herb was thought to ward off evil spirits and to be an elixir of youth and life. I often use rosemary in skin toners for its refreshing and invigorating qualities.

SCENT
Piercing, fresh, herbaceous

NOTE

| BASE | MIDDLE | TOP |

EXPENSE RATING
*

CAUTIONS
Avoid in pregnancy, high blood pressure and epilepsy. See page 16.

Main constituents: pinene, cineol, camphor, camphene, bornyl acetate, borneol

---

THERAPEUTIC PROPERTIES

Traditionally rosemary was used as a fumigant for sick rooms and to protect against infectious disease. It was also known for its invigorating, uplifting qualities. Research in Germany in 1987 found that the herb has a stimulating effect on the central nervous system, which supports claims made by Culpeper and Gerard.

EMOTIONS & MIND
Invigorating and stimulating. Use for massaging the face and head (see pages 98–99).

ACHES & PAINS
Stimulates the skin to boost circulation and ease pain. For rheumatic aches, use in massage oil; if joint is inflamed, omit massage and use a compress instead (see pages 100–1).

RESPIRATORY PROBLEMS
The scent eases cold symptoms and clears congestion. Put two drops on a handkerchief and inhale or massage the chest with diluted oil.

FRESH FLOWERING tops from Mediterranean countries are used to make top quality oil.

LEG MASSAGE

The stimulating action of rosemary oil eases aches (see pages 64–65).

DIGESTIVE PROBLEMS
Relieves headaches that are related to indigestion (see pages 104–5).

ALLERGIES & INFECTIONS
Anti-fungal, anti-bacterial. Use as a disinfectant to help prevent infection and deodorize the air (see page 97).

SKIN & BEAUTY
Rosemary has a refreshing, invigorating effect on the skin, and is an effective addition to any toner (see page 72). After washing hair, add to the final rinse to stimulate the scalp, increase shine and clear dandruff.

OIL COMBINATIONS

Juniper

Lemon-grass

Petitgrain

THE HEALING PROPERTIES OF ROSEMARY are enhanced when blended with lemon-grass and juniper for muscular aches. Lemon-grass and petitgrain, like all citrus-scented oils, soften the aroma.

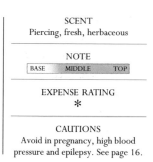

Salvia sclarea
CLARY SAGE

*T*o the Romans, clary sage was a cure-all; the Latin name means "to save". I grow this beautiful herb in my garden, and it gives off a sweet, heady aroma that some people find intoxicating. I often use the essential oil on clients who are convalescing after being in hospital — it is a powerful relaxant with a warm aroma that promotes a sense of well-being.

SCENT
Warm, nutty, herbaceous

NOTE		
BASE	MIDDLE	TOP

EXPENSE RATING
✳✳

CAUTIONS
Avoid in pregnancy; may cause vivid dreams; avoid alcohol. See page 16.

Main constituents: linalyl acetate, linalol, pinene, myrcene, sclareol

THERAPEUTIC PROPERTIES
Essential oil from this plant, which is cultivated in France and Russia, does not share the potential toxicity of essential oil of sage. Both Culpeper and Gerard commented on its use as a remedy for inflammation and noted its ability to bring on menstruation. My clients have also observed these properties, as have midwives, who have used the oil to hasten birth. Clary sage should be avoided in pregnancy until labour. It is also an extremely potent sedative, but in high doses can leave one feeling almost stupefied.

EMOTIONS & MIND
Promotes drowsiness; its euphoric effects are often reflected in an immense sense of well-being. To treat depression or nervous exhaustion, use diluted oil in a slow, soporific back massage or in the bath.

RESPIRATORY PROBLEMS
To ease sore throats, put a couple of drops on a handkerchief and inhale.

GYNAECOLOGICAL PROBLEMS
Anti-spasmodic, warming, analgesic. Excellent for relieving period pains: use in a warm compress (see pages 106–7) or a gentle abdomen massage.

CLARY SAGE OIL is extracted through steam distillation of the leaves and flowering tops of the plant.

SKIN & BEAUTY
Widely used in perfumery. The nutty aroma appeals to men and blends with other warm scents. Use in toners and massage oils (see pages 71–72).

ABDOMEN MASSAGE

The anti-spasmodic properties of clary sage relieve cramps (see pages 62–63).

OIL COMBINATIONS

Melissa

Petitgrain

Rose

MELISSA AND PETITGRAIN enhance the sedative, powerfully relaxing properties of clary sage oil, while rose oil strengthens its uplifting, anti-depressant quality.

Santalum album
SANDALWOOD

*M*entioned in the Nirkuta, *the oldest of the Hindu Vedas (written from the 5th century BC), sandalwood was used in religious ceremonies and plays a key role in Indian Ayurvedic medicine. It is widely used in perfumery for its base note and classic, oriental scent. It is one of my favourite oils; nearly everyone loves its warm, exotic perfume and I use it to calm and pamper my clients.*

SCENT
Sweet, woody, balsamic

NOTE
BASE · MIDDLE · TOP

EXPENSE RATING
✳ ✳ ✳

CAUTIONS
See page 16.

Main constituent: santalol

THERAPEUTIC PROPERTIES

Sandalwood is used to calm and cool the body, reduce inflammation, infection and fever, and to ease sunstroke. I was introduced to it when travelling in India, where 70% of the world's supply is grown (the best oil comes from the Mysore district in south India). An Indian doctor recommended it as the perfect oil for balancing the skin – he used it to soothe inflammation and to calm sensitive, dry, dehydrated skin.

On the last day of the year, it was customary for Burmese women to sprinkle a mixture of sandalwood oil and rose water on those nearby, to wash away the year's sins and purify the body and spirit.

THE HEART WOOD of the tree trunk is used and the oil is extracted from it by steam distillation.

EMOTIONS & MIND
Calming to the mind and emotions; sedative. It enhances the sense of peace that occurs during meditation. Use in massage blends or burn the oil in a vaporizer (see page 97) to treat anxiety and depression.

RESPIRATORY PROBLEMS
Sandalwood oil is used to treat laryngitis, sore throats, bronchitis and chest tightness. Put a couple of drops of oil on a handkerchief and inhale, or massage the area with diluted oil.

URINARY PROBLEMS
Gently antiseptic and diuretic. Useful to treat cystitis. Use sandalwood oil in a warm compress or diluted in a bath or massage blend for the lower back.

ALLERGIES & INFECTIONS
In a French study carried out in 1993, santalol, sandalwood oil's main constituent, was found to be effective in helping to treat gonorrhoea.

SKIN & BEAUTY
Soothing, anti-inflammatory. The oil is beneficial to acne, eczema and chapped, dry skin (see pages 108–9) and is popular in beauty products for its sweet, long-lasting fragrance.

FACIAL MASSAGE

Add sandalwood oil to a pampering massage blend (see pages 80–83).

OIL COMBINATIONS

Jasmine · Frankincense · Rose

IN INDIA, SANDALWOOD is blended with jasmine and frankincense to increase its exotic aroma, and with rose to help create a harmonious scent.

OTHER USEFUL ESSENTIAL OILS

ESSENTIAL OIL	SCENT	NOTE	EXPENSE RATING	SOURCE & EXTRACTION
Styrax benzoin **BENZOIN**	*Sweet, balsamic, warm, vanilla-like*	Base: strong Middle: strong Top: mild	*	Oil is extracted from the gum using solvent. Cultivated in Southeast Asia.
Piper nigrum **BLACK PEPPER**	*Warm, spicy, peppery*	Base: weak Middle: strong Top: strong	**	Oil is extracted from the berries (dried peppercorns) by steam distillation. Cultivated in India, Sri Lanka, Indonesia, Malaysia.
Cedrus atlantica **CEDARWOOD**	*Woody – like a freshly sharpened pencil*	Base: strong Middle: strong Top: weak	*	Oil is extracted from the wood by steam distillation. Cultivated in the Atlas mountains of Morocco.
Zingiber officinale **GINGER**	*Spicy, fresh, camphor-like*	Base: strong Middle: strong Top: mild	*	Oil is extracted from dried, unpeeled rhizome by steam distillation. Cultivated in China and India.
Citrus limonum **LEMON**	*Refreshing, clean, lively*	Base: weak Middle: weak Top: strong	*	Oil is expressed from the peel of fruit. Cultivated in the Mediterranean and North America.
Citrus reticulata **MANDARIN**	*Light, fresh, fruity, popular with children and older people*	Base: weak Middle: weak Top: strong	*	Oil is expressed from the peel of fruit. Cultivated in the Mediterranean, Middle East, Europe, and North and South America.
Pogostemon patchouli **PATCHOULI**	*Very intense, woody, sweet, balsamic*	Base: strong Middle: strong Top: mild	*	Oil is extracted from the dried leaves by steam distillation. Cultivated in South-east Asia, India and the West Indies.
Pinus sylvestris **SCOT'S PINE**	*Medicinal, turpentine-like, balsamic*	Base: weak Middle: weak Top: strong	*	Oil is extracted from the needles and cones by steam distillation. Cultivated in Finland, Norway and Siberia.
Vetiveria zizanoides **VETIVER**	*Rich, warm, smoky, woody, popular with men*	Base: strong Middle: strong Top: mild	**	Oil is extracted from the roots of the grass by steam distillation. Cultivated in India, the Comoro Islands, Haiti and Réunion.
Canaga odorata **YLANG YLANG**	*Heady, floral, tenacious, exotic*	Base: mild Middle: strong Top: strong	**	Oil is extracted from the flowers by steam distillation. Cultivated in the Comoro Islands, Madagascar and Réunion.

Main Constituents	Therapeutic Properties	Common Uses	Cautions (see page 16)
Vanillin, benzoic acid	*Warming and soothing; expectorant; promotes skin healing*	• In inhalations for respiratory problems • Ingredient in hand creams to help heal dry, cracked skin	• May sensitize skin due to solvent extraction • Avoid on babies
Pinene, piperine, limonene, sabinene	*Stimulates blood flow to the skin, therefore warming*	• In massage blends to warm before sport and to prevent stiffness afterward • In abdominal massage blends to combat digestive problems and constipation	• May irritate skin • Use low or very low dilutions (1% or less)
Cedrene, atlantone, cedrol, cadinene	*Stimulating; antiseptic; a general tonic*	• Ingredient in preparations for oily skin • In compresses to relieve rashes and itching • In scalp massage blends to combat dandruff and hair loss	• May irritate and sensitize skin • Use low or very low dilutions (1% or less) • Avoid in pregnancy
Gingerin, gingerol, zingerone, zingiberene, linalol, camphene	*Warming and stimulating*	• In chest rubs for respiratory problems • In massage blends for muscular aches • In compresses for arthritic or inflamed joints and bruises	• May sensitize skin • Use low dilutions (1%) • Avoid on face and neck, and on babies and children
Limonene, pinene, citral, bergaptene, camphene	*Cleansing and refreshing; antiseptic and astringent; a tonic*	• Ingredient in toners for greasy or acne-prone skin • In vaporizers to refresh	• Avoid steam inhalations, sun and sunbeds for 6 hours • Use low dilutions (1%)
Citral, limonene, geraniol, methyl anthranilate	*Calming, refreshing and uplifting; a tonic*	• In massage blends for nervous tension • In compresses for rheumatic aches • In massage blends to help relieve fluid retention and cellulite	• Avoid sun and sunbeds for 6 hours
Patchoulol, patchoulene	*Anti-inflammatory and bactericidal; a tonic; said to be an aphrodisiac*	• In massage blends for skin conditions, such as acne and eczema, and for ageing skin, dandruff and greasy hair	• May cause headaches
Monoterpenes, bornyl acetate, cadinene, pinene, sylvestrene	*Invigorating; antiseptic; stimulates blood flow to the skin, therefore warming*	• In inhalations for coughs, colds, catarrh and sinus congestion • In massage blends for stiffness and aches • In vaporizers to fight airborne microbes	• May irritate skin • Use low or very low dilutions (1% or less)
Vetiverol, vitivone, terpenes	*Strong sedative; calming; antiseptic*	• In massage blends for insomnia • In compresses for acne • Ingredient in aftershave lotions	• Strong sedative; avoid if driving • Often adulterated
Linalol, geraniol, pinene, benzyl acetate	*Sedative; euphoric*	• In massage blends for stress • Ingredient in perfumes and hair- and skin-care preparations • Ingredient in pampering bath products	• May cause headaches and nausea • Use low dilutions (1%)

MASSAGE TECHNIQUES

My personal motto is "life takes it out of you, but massage puts it back". The basis of massage is touch and, to thrive, we all need the warmth and security it engenders. On the following pages I demonstrate all the basic massage strokes and show how to combine them in a relaxing full body massage.

PREPARING TO MASSAGE

A massage with scented oil blends should be as relaxing to give as it is to receive, with one movement flowing into the next, leaving you and your partner calm. As with any new skill, massage takes practice. Try to persuade a friend to learn as well, so that you can massage each other and appreciate how the strokes feel. During a massage, it is essential that both you and your partner feel at ease, so start by making your environment as comfortable as possible.

ENVIRONMENT

Choose a peaceful, quiet, warm room with subdued lighting. I like to work on the floor, padded with a futon or a couple of thick blankets, as it provides plenty of space to spread out. To prevent sore knees, kneel on a cushion and change your position often. You can also work on a sturdy, well-padded kitchen table, or you may wish to invest in a massage couch, especially if you tend to get a tired back or if kneeling for prolonged periods causes you discomfort. Most traditional beds are too soft for massage and absorb all your strength. Cover the table or floor with towels. I place a small electric blanket or hot water bottle under the towels, and the gentle heat keeps my clients warm.

YOUR COMFORT

Wear loose, comfortable clothing, remove jewellery, and make sure your nails are short. To give a good massage, you need to be absorbed in what you are doing. Concentrate on your friend, breathe deeply, and enjoy the rhythm of the movements – your sense of tranquillity will be transmitted to your friend. Keep your back as straight as possible during the massage, and use your body weight, instead of force, to vary the depth of the movements. Learn to be sensitive and to "listen" with your hands. To increase flexibility, squeeze a rubber ball in each hand, flexing and extending your fingers for a minute a day.

PAMPERING YOUR FRIEND

Your friend's general health and what he or she hopes to gain from the massage will govern your choice of essential oils. For instance, is stress a problem? Does your friend need to feel wide awake at the end of the treatment, or is there time to sleep afterward? Discuss contraindications (see Warnings below), and then select an appropriate blend of essential oils from pages 17–39, ensuring that he or she likes the aroma. Once your friend has undressed, cover the body with plenty of large towels to keep in warmth and enhance the feeling of comfort. It is surprising how cold one can become just lying still, and this makes it impossible to relax.

WARNINGS

Before starting to massage, ask whether your friend is pregnant or epileptic, and if so, see the advice on page 16.

Never massage someone with any of the following conditions without a doctor's consent:

- Inflammatory conditions, such as varicose veins, thrombosis or phlebitis
- Acute back pain, especially if the pain shoots down the arms or legs when you touch the back
- Skin infection, bruising or acute inflammation
- Infection, contagious disease or high temperature
- Any other serious medical condition.

USING MASSAGE OIL

Oil helps the hands glide smoothly over the body. For a full body massage, you will need about 20 ml (4 tsp) of carrier oil, to which you can add a few drops of essential oil (see page 15). The amount of oil you use will depend on the size of your friend and the dryness of the skin. Shake the bottle, then warm a little oil between your hands. Keep the open bottle within reach in case you need to apply more oil. If you do, keep one hand on the body while picking up the bottle.

APPLYING THE OIL

Pour about a teaspoon of oil into the palm of one hand (not over the fingers – it will drip through), warm it between your palms, then stroke it on to the body. Never pour oil directly on to the skin.

TO REPLENISH THE OIL, drizzle a small amount on to the back of your hand and use your other hand to stroke the oil on to the body

BASIC MASSAGE STROKES

Once you have mastered the basic strokes, you can use them all over the body and tailor each massage to suit the individual needs of your partner. Before you start practising a new movement, read through the instructions and concentrate on learning just a few strokes at a time. To avoid awkward twisting, face the area you are massaging, and keep your back as straight as possible. Direct your strokes toward the heart, using your body weight to add depth.

FAN STROKING

Stroking movements are among the easiest and most calming to give and receive in massage, and you will probably return to them often to calm your friend and relax yourself. Use Fan Stroking to apply oil and to link different areas of the body, and when your hands are tired or you are deciding which movement to use next. Work smoothly and rhythmically. You can vary the length of the stroke, but keep the rhythm fluid.

1 Place your hands side by side on the body, palms down, and then smoothly and gently glide upward, leading with your fingers. Keeping your back straight, lean forward on to your hands, using the weight of your body to apply a steady, even pressure through the palms and heels of the hands.

2 Fan your hands out to both sides of the body, reducing the pressure, and slide them down the sides, moulding them to the contours of the body. Pull your hands up toward each other, and swivel them around to begin the upward movement again. Repeat several times, covering the whole area.

ALTERNATE FAN STROKING

Follow the sequence above, using each hand alternately to stroke the body. This slight variation creates wonderful diagonal stretches. Starting with the right hand, stroke firmly upward and out. Then repeat the movement with the left hand so that it strokes up as the right hand glides down. Repeat several times to cover the whole area.

CIRCULAR STROKING

In this variation of Fan Stroking, both hands work on the same side, one hand completing a full circle while the other makes a half circle, building up a smooth and steady rhythm. Circular Stroking is particularly effective on large areas, such as the back, shoulders and abdomen and, like Fan Stroking, is good for linking different areas in a full body massage. It produces a continuous flowing effect.

1 Place both hands, fingers pointing away from you, on one side of the body about 15 cm (6 in) apart.

2 △ Start to circle your hands in a clockwise direction, starting with the left hand and following with the right.

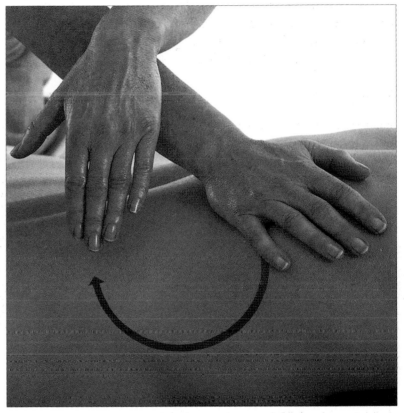

3 △ As your left hand meets your right arm, lift it over, rejoining the body on the other side to complete the circle.

Repeat several times, stroking firmly on the upward and outward movement, and gliding gently to complete the circle.

THUMB STROKING

This firm movement is particularly useful on small, tense areas, such as the top of the shoulders and the neck. Alter the pressure to suit your friend's needs. If the muscles are very tight, begin gently, then stroke more firmly. To vary the effect, circle your thumbs, following steps 1–3 above for Circular Stroking.

With your hands resting on the body, stroke firmly upward and out to the side with your left thumb. Follow with the right thumb, stroking a little higher. Make the stroke smooth and repetitive, building up a steady rhythm.

BASIC KNEADING

In a relaxing massage, kneading should be flat and smooth to produce an amazingly soothing effect. The movement is like kneading dough, and is useful on the shoulders, back and fleshy areas such as the hips. In Sarawak, Malaysia, on the island of Borneo, I learned to appreciate how soporific kneading can be when performed rhythmically. Normala, a Malaysian physiotherapist, taught me the value of counting "and one, and two, and three, and four, and five" over and over as I slowly kneaded. The monotony is very calming.

1 Place your hands flat on the body with your elbows apart, and fingers pointing away from you. With your right hand, gently grasp some flesh and release it into your left hand.

2 Let your left hand take the flesh and then release it into your right hand. Repeat several times, counting to keep your strokes rhythmic, like waves washing over the muscles.

CIRCULAR PRESSURES

Deep, penetrating circles are useful for exploring the state of the muscles, and for combating tension. Apply the pressure gradually, beginning to circle more deeply and firmly, then slowly release and move on to the next area. For tight, knotted muscles, place one thumb on top of the other, and lean into the body.

Using only a small amount of oil — too much will cause your thumbs to slide — place the pads of your thumbs on the skin and gradually lean into them. Press for a few seconds, then make small, penetrating, circular movements against the underlying muscle. Glide to the next area, and repeat the movement.

STATIC PRESSURES

Stationary pressure is extremely useful for releasing tension in the neck and shoulders, sides of the spine, buttocks and soles of the feet. Ease into the pressure gradually and steadily, hold, and then slowly release — never poke sharply. Treat the body with care, making sure that your fingernails do not gouge the skin.

For this movement no oil is necessary. Place the pads of your thumbs on the skin and gradually lean into them. Hold for 5—9 seconds, then release slowly and glide to the next point of tension. Imagine how it feels to receive the massage — this helps your hands respond to the area you are working on.

KNUCKLING

For a heavenly sensation, rotate your knuckles on the shoulders, chest, palms of the hands, soles of the feet, and hips. You can work deeply without hurting.

Curl your hands into loose fists and, with the middle section of your fingers against the skin, ripple your fingers around in small, circular movements. Vary the pressure by leaning into the movement with more or less body weight. Work firmly and evenly to cover the whole of a tense area.

CAT STROKING

This is one of the nicest strokes with which to finish massaging an area. If done slowly and rhythmically it can soon send the recipient to sleep. Use a soft, gentle touch, and keep your movements smooth.

Place your left hand at the top of the area you are massaging and stroke slowly and lightly down the body, as if stroking a cat. Lift it off at the bottom of the area and return it to the start while the right hand begins the downward stroke. Repeat, making the return movement as smooth as the stroking.

HOLDING

Many people love just being held – especially on the head, forehead and abdomen. Simple holds are relaxing, comforting, and as calming for the person giving the massage as for the recipient.

Place one hand over the other, and gently hold. Concentrate on your partner's breathing and relax, releasing very slowly after one or two minutes. Never hurry this movement at the end of a massage: its effect will remain long after the massage finishes. If time is short, omit an earlier stroke rather than rushing this hold.

A FULL BODY MASSAGE

Massaging the whole body with aromatic oils has the power to release muscular tension, increase energy and create a feeling of well-being. This massage starts on the back, moves down to the feet, and then continues on the front from head to toes. It takes about an hour and a half. Before you begin, discuss your friend's health to ensure that massage is safe (see page 42). Ask her to remove make-up, jewellery and contact lenses. Remind her that she is in charge and must say if she feels uncomfortable.

THE BACK

EVERYBODY LOVES A BACK MASSAGE and, as most of the basic movements are used here, it is an ideal place to start. I begin by slowly stroking down the back to enhance relaxation. Work smoothly and rhythmically to create a hypnotic effect. If your hands get tired as you massage or you aren't sure what to do next, just stroke.

STARTING THE MASSAGE

1 *Kneel by your friend's left side. Place your left hand over the towel at the top of the back, and your right hand over the small of the back. Hold, breathing slowly to relax yourself and your friend.*

2 ◁ *Place your right hand on the left shoulder blade, and your left hand on the right hip. Lean forward to gently stretch the back. Repeat on the other side.*

WHOLE BACK STROKING

Choose an appropriate blend of essential oils (see pages 18–39) and mix them in a carrier oil.

1 ▽ *Fold the towel down. Sitting behind your friend's head, apply about a teaspoon of oil, as shown on page 43. Only apply more oil if your hands drag the skin. Place one hand on either side of the spine at the top of the back and stroke down the back extremely slowly as far as you can reach.*

2 *At the base of the spine, fan your hands out over the hips, and mould them around the sides of the back as you glide up to the shoulders and around the tops of the arms.*

3 *Press down slightly as your hands swivel around the shoulders, before stroking smoothly down the back again, on either side of the spine. Repeat steps 1–3 several times to give your friend a wonderful, all-engulfing sensation.*

KEEP YOUR BACK STRAIGHT — the more comfortable and relaxed you are, the better your massage will be

KNEELING BEHIND your friend's head allows you to direct your strokes downward

4 *Starting at the shoulders, let both hands simultaneously fan out from either side of the spine and glide back (see Fan Stroking, page 44). With each movement, fan your hands out a little lower, going as far down the back as you can reach. Vary the stroke by alternating your hands to give the back a lovely diagonal stretch.*

5 *Working away from the spine on one side of the back, then the other, let one hand complete a full circle, and the other a half circle (see Circular Stroking, page 45). Circle continuously, moulding your hands to the body's contours.*

FIGURES OF EIGHT

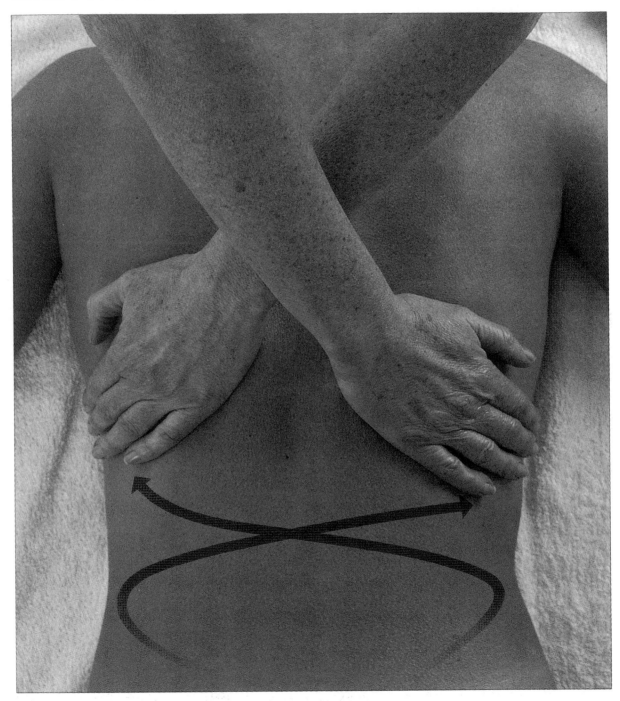

1 This relaxing stroke is a favourite with my clients. With one hand on each side of the spine at shoulder-level, stroke firmly down to the small of the back. Fan out over the hips.

2 △ Now glide back up, criss-crossing the body to form a series of figures of eight. Pull up at the sides and release as you cross the spine — never press on the spine. Repeat three times.

WORKING MORE DEEPLY

1 Stroking with one thumb following the other, work down the right side of the neck and out to the top of the shoulder, keeping the movement firm to release taut muscles and ease away tension. Repeat on the left side.

2 Make large, flat circles with your thumbs on either side of the spine, from the shoulders down to the small of the back. Alter the depth and size of the circles: smaller, deeper circles are more penetrating and effective on tense areas.

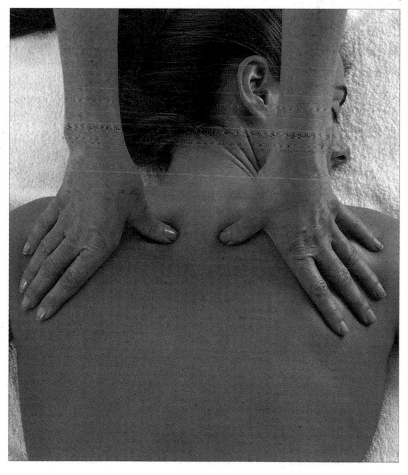

3 △ Now place both thumbs on the right side of the spine by the shoulder. Make a full circle with one thumb and a half circle with the other, stroking away from the spine and working as far down the back as you can reach. This motion is similar to Circular Stroking (see page 45). Repeat on the left side.

4 ▷ Use Static Pressures (see page 46) on either side of the spine, from the base of the neck to the pelvis, on the tops of the shoulders and into the scalp. Slowly lean on to your thumbs, hold the pressure for 5–9 seconds, and release. Work slowly and carefully, using less weight on the neck, the base of the skull and scalp.

UNDULATING STROKES

1 *Rhythmically knead the upper arms, shoulders and back (see page 46). With alternate hands slowly grasp and release the flesh, like kneading dough. Do five sets of five strokes on each area, counting to yourself to keep the rhythm. Knead the neck with thumbs and fingers.*

2 *◁ Roll your middle knuckles around the top and sides of the shoulders, the base of the spine, and out over the hips (see page 47). This deep yet relaxing movement feels heavenly.*

3 *Pick up some flesh to the right of the base of the spine and roll it between your thumbs and fingers up the back. I call this the inchworm. Repeat on the left.*

KNUCKLING ALLOWS you to work deeply on tense areas without hurting

FINISHING TOUCHES

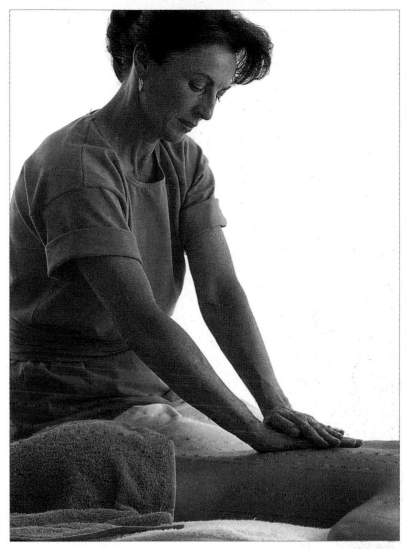

1 Place your left hand over your right to the right of the base of the spine, and make large, sweeping circles away from the spine up to the shoulder. Circle around the shoulder, relax the pressure and glide down to the lower left side. Then circle up the left side. Repeat several times. Then circle around the hips.

2 ▷ Keeping your left hand over your right, stiffen your arms and tense the muscles so that your hands vibrate gently as you stroke (without pressure) down from the top of the spine to its base. This small movement may take practice, but it is incredibly relaxing. Repeat twice.

3 Place your right hand on the neck, fingers pointing toward the head, and in a smooth, slow movement bring it down the spine and smoothly lift it off at the base as your left hand gently repeats the stroke. This hypnotic movement will make your partner feel like a stroked cat.

4 Rest your forearms horizontally across the middle of the back, with your wrists relaxed, and gradually stroke outward, your left arm going toward the head and your right arm toward the legs. Lean into this lovely long stretch.

5 Cover your friend with a towel and finish the back massage with smooth rocking. With your left hand, hold the shoulder while your right hand gently rocks the small of the back to and fro. My clients frequently say this takes them back to their childhood and gives them a sense of security and peace.

THE BACK OF THE LEGS & FEET

FOLLOWING THE BACK MASSAGE, move down the body to begin work on the back of the legs and feet. Keep the rest of your friend's body covered with towels so that she stays warm while you massage first one leg, then the other. The movements described here help to relieve tension and dispel fatigue while stimulating the circulation, and many of them can also be used on the front of the legs (see pages 64–65).

UPPER LEG STROKES

Apply a teaspoon of oil initially, adding more as necessary to keep your movements smooth.

1 Kneel by the right foot. Apply some oil and place your left hand on the inner side of the right calf, your right hand on the outer side. Stroke both hands firmly up the leg, spreading the oil. Glide back down – at the calf let one hand slide under the leg, the other over the back of it.

2 Now kneel by your friend's right side, facing the thigh. Try to keep one hand in contact with the body while you move. Knead the thigh in rows (see page 46), keeping your hands open and relaxed. Count as you knead to maintain the rhythm.

3 ◁ Place your left hand on the inner thigh and your right hand on the outer thigh, and bring your hands together, pulling the flesh up toward the top of the leg. Release, then bring the flesh up from the other side, criss-crossing the leg.

4 Gently circle the thumbs of both hands over the back of the knee, without applying pressure. Gentle massage here is very soothing and helps to stimulate the lymphatic system, which cleanses the body and returns water and proteins to the blood.

LOWER LEG STROKES

1 Kneeling by your friend's feet, bend her right leg and rest the foot on your shoulder. Stroke from the ankle toward the knee with your palms, then knead the calf with alternating hands.

2 ▷ Stroke down the calf from ankle to knee with your right, then left forearm, and glide back. Repeat several times.

3 Lower the leg and circle your thumbs rhythmically around the ankle. Stroke the sole of the foot with your thumbs, and then circle around the heel.

4 Press the middle knuckles of both hands into the sole of the foot as if walking on it. Repeat three times. Then relax your friend by sandwiching the foot between your hands. Repeat the entire massage sequence on the left leg.

THE FACE

WHILE YOUR FRIEND TURNS over and settles under the towels, wash your hands and double check that she has removed contact lenses. This simple face massage should only take about 15 minutes. Although it is easier to work with oil or cream, it is possible to do the massage without any lubricant if your partner doesn't want her hair to get oily. If you prefer, you can do this massage at the end of the full body massage.

Use just enough oil to allow your hands to move freely without slipping over the skin.

1 Sit behind your friend's head. If you use oil, apply it with your palms from the forehead to the neck. Then stroke out from the centre of the brow to the temples. Repeat three times.

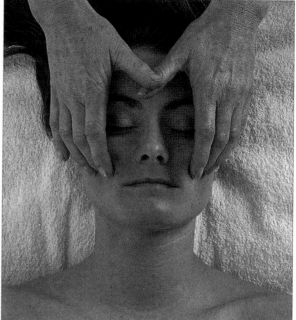

2 Using your thumbs, stroke from the centre of the forehead out to the temples, working first at the hairline, then on the middle of the forehead and, finally, on the eyebrows. Repeat the movement three times, gently stroking away tension.

3 With your thumbs, stroke from the forehead down the bridge of the nose, under the cheekbones, and up to the temples. Then apply gentle pressure with two fingers beside the nostrils, under the cheekbones, and at the temples. Repeat three times.

4 Stroke your left hand, then your right hand, up the neck, from the left shoulder to the ear. Repeat six times, then work on the right side.

5 △ Sandwich the jaw between your fingers and thumbs, and gently stroke out from the chin to the ear with alternate hands. Repeat six times.

6 Place your middle fingers between the eyebrows. In a circular movement, stroke out firmly over the brows, and in gently under the eyes. Repeat six times.

7 ▷ Stroke your palms and fingers slowly up the forehead into the hair. Then place your palms on the forehead and hold for about a minute to create a feeling of security and calmness.

REST YOUR HANDS on the forehead, feeling the rhythm of your friend's breathing

CHEST, SHOULDERS & NECK

ALMOST EVERYONE CARRIES TENSION in the shoulders and neck, so this is an extremely popular area to massage. By working on the chest, you relax the muscles and encourage deeper breathing. With your partner lying on her back you can easily get your fingers behind the neck to massage either side of the spine and work on the base of the skull. As you use these gentle, hypnotic strokes, tension will melt away.

1 Kneel behind your friend's head and begin by massaging over the towel that covers her. Imagine that the heels of your hands are a cat's paws and "walk" over the chest. This rhythmic movement will help her to relax.

Pour a small amount of oil into your palm, and remember to rub your hands together to warm it.

2 ▷ Fold down the towel. Apply some oil to your hands and place them on the collar bone; fan firmly out over the top of the chest and shoulders and gently push down, releasing as you complete the circle. Now circle out over the shoulders. Repeat six times.

3 △ Rest your forearms on the floor and loosely rotate your fingers against the base of the neck, using your knuckles to loosen taut muscles. Anyone with tense shoulders will love this movement.

4 Stroke your hands up the back of the neck, and pull gently at the base of the skull to stretch the neck slightly. Release, and repeat the movement at least four times.

5 Stroke your thumbs out from the centre of the chest, just below the collar bone, along the muscles between the ribs. Repeat the movement as far down as it is comfortable for your friend, avoiding the breasts. Ask your friend to tell you if she feels any discomfort.

6 ▷ Rest the head on your left hand. Stroke your right hand down the back of the neck to the shoulder and repeat several times. Make deep circles on this side of the spine, back of the neck and shoulder. Repeat on the other side.

7 Cup your hands behind the neck. Gently take the weight of the head in your hands. Slowly and carefully stretch it toward you.

8 Support the skull with your fingers while your palms cup the ears, blocking out extraneous noise. Hold, concentrating on your friend's breathing.

ARMS & HANDS

TENSION IN ONE AREA can often be released by stroking another part of the body, which is one of the reasons a complete body massage is so relaxing. If tense arms are causing the shoulders to ache, these calm, hypnotic movements will soothe, and gently ease tension out of the muscles. Arm muscles are usually strong, so your movements here can be firm, while simply holding and stroking the hand can be calming and reassuring to your massage partner.

LEAN INTO the stroke, keeping your back straight

MASSAGING THE ARMS

Apply a small amount of oil to your hands if they are not moving smoothly over the skin.

1 Kneel by your friend's left side. Support the elbow with your left hand; stroke your right hand around the arm, back of the shoulder and neck. Repeat three times.

2 ◁ Still supporting the elbow, knead the upper arm with your right hand (see page 46). Repeat six times, changing hands to cover the arm. Knead the top of the shoulder and back of the neck.

3 ◁ Place your left hand above the left shoulder, and slide your right hand underneath the body, hooking your fingers around the shoulder blade. Guide with your left hand while your right hand gently pulls toward you, stretching the muscles.

4 Stroke the entire arm, including the elbow. Support the wrist with your left hand, and with your right hand knead the lower arm slowly. Change hands to cover the whole area.

STROKING THE HANDS

1 *Explore the wrist with your thumbs, being aware of its eight small bones.*

2 ▷ *Support your friend's hand with your fingers while your thumbs stroke up from the base of the fingers over the back of the hand to the wrist. Repeat with one thumb following the other.*

3 *Hold your friend's hand, palm down, in your left hand. With your right hand, squeeze all over each finger from the base to the fingertip. Then gently rotate each finger twice in each direction. Smoothly and gently pull each finger, taking care not to jerk the joints.*

4 *Support the back of your friend's hand with your left hand while your right palm strokes her palm.*

5 *Placing her hand between yours, rotate the heels of your hands over and around her knuckles to loosen them.*

6 ▷ *Sandwich your partner's hand between your own hands and draw away slowly. Repeat several times before releasing. Repeat the entire arm and hand massage on the right side.*

THE ABDOMEN

GREAT SENSITIVITY IS REQUIRED when massaging the abdomen because many people are nervous about being touched here. Reassure your friend that your strokes will be gentle, and massage confidently in a clockwise direction, following the workings of the intestines. Smooth, repetitive massage with aromatic oils helps to calm the nerves, combat constipation and stimulate the digestive system while toning the skin.

1 Kneel by your friend's right side, facing the abdomen. Place your hands gently over the towels covering her, and slowly rock her abdomen back and forth to loosen the muscles and ease tension.

 Pour about a teaspoon of oil into your palm, and rub your hands together to warm it.

2 ▷ Fold back the towels and apply some oil. Lightly rest your left hand on the rib cage or just below it, and with your right hand circle the navel in a clockwise direction. Circle smoothly and confidently, gradually getting firmer and building a steady rhythm. Then gently introduce the left hand to the stroke, so that both hands are circling the navel (see Circular Stroking, page 45). Stroke continuously, feeling the tension abate.

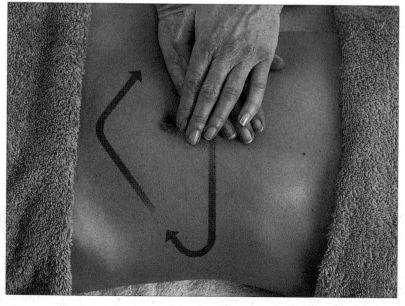

3 ◁ With your left hand on your right, make an undulating movement, gently pressing and releasing as you work in a triangle around the navel. Keep the movement fluid and rhythmic.

4 With flat, open hands, knead the far side of the abdomen, followed by the middle section, and then the near side (see page 46). Count while you knead to keep the rhythm constant.

5 ▽ *Place both hands below the navel, pointing upward, and stroke up the abdomen and out over the ribs. Glide down the sides of the body, slide your hands under the back, and pull up at the waist (but not if your friend is larger than you).*

6 *Ask your friend to raise her back and slide your hands beneath it. Firmly circle your fingers beside the spine, working against the weight of the body for added depth.*

7 *Cup your hands over the navel. Hold for a few seconds, then gently vibrate on the area before slowly releasing.*

RAISE ONE LEG
to support
your back

GENTLY PULLING up
at the waist releases
pent-up tension

THE FRONT OF THE LEGS

WHEN MASSAGING THE LEG, imagine that you are sculpting it into a perfect shape – this will help your strokes to go in the right direction. Begin on the left leg, and continue with the foot massage shown on pages 66–67 before returning to massage the right leg. These firm, repetitive movements stimulate the circulation, dispel fatigue, help to relieve aches and pains, and can also be used before or after exercise.

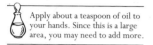

Apply about a teaspoon of oil to your hands. Since this is a large area, you may need to add more.

1 Kneel by the left foot and apply some oil to your hands. Place your left hand under the left foot, your right hand on top, sandwiching it. Slide slowly and firmly up the leg and glide down. Repeat several times, building up a rhythm.

2 Kneel beside the left leg. With alternate hands, knead the thigh by methodically squeezing and releasing the flesh. Use firm strokes on the outer thigh and gentle strokes on the inner thigh.

LEAN INTO this simple but strong movement, using your body weight to add depth

3 Place one hand on either side of the thigh, fingers facing away from you, and firmly bring your hands toward each other. Release them on top of the leg and glide down the other side in a criss-cross movement. Repeat six times.

4 Knuckle the thigh with both hands (see page 47), paying special attention to the outer thigh.

5 ▷ Keeping a V-shaped space between your index finger and thumb, stroke your left hand firmly up the thigh then lift off to start again while your right hand begins the stroke. Repeat six times.

6 *Kneel by your friend's left calf. Place your left hand under the knee while your right palm and thumb circle around the kneecap.*

7 *Support the ankle with your left hand. Slowly and smoothly stroke and knead the calf with your right hand. Swap hands to cover the whole area.*

LEAD WITH your left arm up the thigh, making the stroke long and smooth

8 *Circle your fingers around the ankles, then stroke your hands up the muscles on either side of the calf to encourage lymph flow (see page 88). Glide down and repeat six times.*

THE FEET

MASSAGING THE FOOT with scented oils can be particularly relaxing and usually evokes sighs of delight. It relieves fatigue, and revitalizes and relaxes the whole body. Because some people are ticklish on their feet and may be nervous at first, use confident, firm movements with just enough oil to allow your fingers to move smoothly.

Apply a small amount of oil – too much will cause your fingers to slip and slide.

1 Kneel in front of your friend's left foot. Apply a little oil to your hands. Supporting the foot with the fingers of both hands, stroke your thumbs from the base of the toes up to the ankle.

KEEP YOUR WRISTS LOOSE — the more relaxed you are, the better the massage will feel

2 Support the foot with your left hand and use your right thumb and index finger to squeeze between the joints of each toe, feeling the underlying structure as you work. Massage each toe individually, gently rolling, rubbing and squeezing it all over, including the nail tip. Then carefully pull each toe toward you, slowly stretching it.

3 Rest your right hand on the top of the foot, and roll and press the knuckles of your left hand into the ball of the foot. Repeat three times.

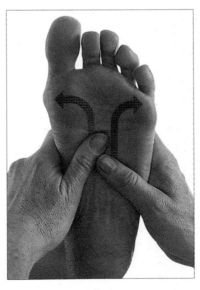

4 Still resting your right hand on top of the foot, stroke the heel of your left hand firmly down from the ball of the foot into the arch and then down to the heel. Repeat three times.

5 ◁ Supporting the foot with your fingers, stroke both thumbs firmly up the sole. At the ball of the foot stroke out in a T-shape, glide back down toward the heel and repeat six times.

6 Sandwich the foot between your hands and stroke several times up toward the body, then slowly draw your hands away. Repeat the sequence on the right leg and foot (return to page 64).

AROMATIC BEAUTY CARE

Avicenna, the 10th-century philosopher and physician, claimed that diet, exercise and sleep were the prerequisites for health. I believe that health and beauty are inextricably linked and that a few minutes' massage each day using the nourishing aromatherapy beauty preparations on the following pages makes skin care a pleasure.

MAKING BEAUTY BASICS

My philosophy for skin care is simple: we do not need hundreds of exotic products, just a few that really work, including a cleanser, toner, moisturizer, mask and massage oil or cream. I will never forget the excitement of making my first cosmetics. The process is as easy as basic cookery. It is also inexpensive and allows you to select essential oils with scents you enjoy and ingredients to suit your skin type. Like food, skin-care products should be prepared under hygienic conditions. If kept in a refrigerator, most should last at least a month.

THE FINISHED PRODUCTS

Cleansing grains

Moisturizing cream

Pomade

Clay mask

Fruit mask

INGREDIENTS & EQUIPMENT

For some recipes, special ingredients and equipment are required in addition to carrier oils (see page 14), essential oils (see pages 17–39) and basic kitchen items.

SPECIAL INGREDIENTS

Fullers earth: an earthy, hydrous aluminium silicate capable of absorbing grease
Green clay: the finest clay, for sensitive and dry skin
Kaolin: a fine white powder with a gentle astringent effect; use for normal or oily skin
Beeswax: a hard, waxy secretion from honeycomb
Lanolin: thick, sticky sebum from sheep's wool with a softening effect; use the anhydrous variety in the recipes

Cocoa butter: a solidified butter-like substance obtained from the roasted cocoa bean
Distilled water: water purified by distillation
Flower water: water infused with flowers

SPECIAL EQUIPMENT

Sterilized dark glass bottles: small (30 ml) and larger (100 ml) for storing oils and toners
Sterilized jars: 30 ml and 100 ml for storing creams, pomades and washing grains

Heat-resistant bowls: small and medium sizes in which to mix ingredients
Funnels: to transfer oil or toner into bottles
Coffee filter paper: for filtering toners

Funnels

Lanolin

Beeswax

Glass jars and bottles

Fullers earth

Green clay

Kaolin

Cocoa butter

Filter paper

UNDERSTANDING YOUR SKIN

Skin, which is your protection against the elements, blocks out bacteria and by perspiring eliminates waste and water. Under perfect conditions, the skin will be self-cleaning, self-lubricating and self-renewing, but sun, wind and harsh products disrupt these natural processes and can cause the following problems.

Dry skin is often fine, delicately textured and can feel as though it is pulled too tightly over the face. It has a tendency to develop broken capillaries and tiny lines which, if neglected, turn into wrinkles. To prevent premature ageing and dehydration, use plenty of rich emollient creams and oils, made with jojoba, avocado and sweet almond carrier oils. Dry skin responds well to essential oils that encourage skin renewal, including benzoin, frankincense, jasmine, lavender, rose and sandalwood.

Oily skin tends to look sallow and greasy and has a heavy, unrefined texture. The grease picks up dirt, clogging the pores, which can lead to blackheads and spots. Keep oily skin meticulously clean: moisturize only where it feels dry, usually avoiding the chin and nose. Use sunflower-, grapeseed- or soya-based creams and oils, containing geranium, bergamot, lavender, rosemary or cypress essential oils for their antiseptic properties.

Combination skin is characterized by dry areas around the cheeks, neck and eyes, and an oily T-shaped panel on the forehead, nose and chin. Balance the two types of skin by moisturizing the dry areas and keeping the oily parts really clean.

Sensitive skin can be of any type, and may become sensitive from rough handling or exposure to harsh products. Treat with simple sweet almond- or jojoba-based oils and creams containing soothing essential oils like chamomile.

Acne is caused by over-active sebaceous glands. Oil build-up blocks hair follicles, producing blackheads, while organisms living on the sebum break down into acids, causing swelling and spots. Treat with diluted tea tree oil (see pages 108–9).

CLEANSING GRAINS

It is important to cleanse the skin gently to remove daily dirt and oil without stripping it of its natural oils. These washing grains have a gentle exfoliating effect and should be used once or twice a week instead of soap. Choose fine oatmeal for a mildly abrasive scrub, or medium oatmeal for a stronger, more abrasive scrub.

HONEY & OATMEAL WASHING GRAINS

Essential oils
12 drops (orange and geranium oils work well)

Base
1 cup oatmeal, fine or medium
$^1\!/_2$ cup ground almonds
10 ml sweet almond oil
1 tbsp clear honey

1 Put the oatmeal and almonds into a medium bowl. Set aside. In a small bowl, mix the oils and honey.

2 △ Add the oil mixture to the dry ingredients, stirring until well-mixed. Transfer to a sterilized jar. To use, moisten a teaspoon of grains with a little rose water and rub gently over face. Rinse off.

AROMATIC OILS

This simple recipe makes a good cleanser, massage oil and bath oil. Adjust the amounts to suit your needs: 5 ml is enough for a bath, 10 ml for the face and 20 ml for a body massage; or make more and store for future use (see page 16).

BASIC OIL

Essential oils
6–10 drops (choose from 3–4 oils)

Carrier oil
20 ml to suit skin type (see above)

Pour the carrier oil through a funnel into a small, dark glass bottle. Add the essential oils, seal and shake well.

VARIATION

Relaxing oil to soothe jangled nerves: add clary sage, marjoram and chamomile to sweet almond oil.

TONERS

Skin toners and aftershave lotions, made by infusing essential oils in distilled water, leave the skin fresh, clean and invigorated.

BASIC TONER

Essential oils
25 drops (choose from up to 4 oils)
Base
100 ml distilled water or flower water

1 Pour the water into a large, sterilized dark bottle. Add the essential oil and allow to stand for a month, shaking often.

2 Pour through a filter paper-lined funnel into a large bottle. Shake.

BASIC AROMATIC VINEGAR

Essential oil
5–6 drops
Base
10 ml wine or cider vinegar, or vodka
80 ml distilled water

1 Pour the alcohol through a funnel into a small, sterilized dark bottle and add the essential oil. Allow to stand for a week, shaking the bottle daily.

2 Pour the toner through filter paper. Dilute with distilled water, and store in a large, sterilized dark bottle.

BASIC HONEY WATER

Essential oils
5 drops
Base
10 ml vodka
¼ tsp honey
80 ml orange flower water

Mix the vodka, honey and oils, and pour into a small, sterilized dark bottle. Allow to stand for ten days, shaking at times. Dilute with water. Store in a larger bottle.

VARIATION

Orange toner: use 10 drops petitgrain, 10 orange and 5 neroli in the basic toner recipe. Dilute with orange flower water.

CREAMS

Made of oils, waxes and water, creams keep the skin pliable while providing protection against the elements. Select creams based on your skin type and preference. I believe that regular massage is the best way to apply cream because it improves circulation and aids absorption. These recipes make about 100 ml, enough to keep.

BASIC CREAM

Essential oil
4–6 drops
Base
7 gm beeswax
60 ml sweet almond oil
30 ml flower water
or distilled water

VARIATIONS

*1 **Light cream**: add 35 ml jojoba in step 1, increase the beeswax to 10 gm, reduce the oil to 45 ml and the water to 20 ml.*
*2 **Rich treatment cream**: add 15 gm lanolin in step 1, reduce the oil to 45 ml and increase the water to 60 ml.*
*3 **Luxurious cream**: add 15 gm cocoa butter in step 1, decrease the oil to 45 ml and increase the water to 35 ml.*

1 Put the beeswax and carrier oil into a heat-resistant bowl. Stir over a pan of boiling water until the mixture melts.

2 Remove the bowl from the pan, and slowly add the water to the mixture, stirring constantly.

3 Keep stirring while the cream begins to cool, then add the essential oil. Stir until the mixture has thickened, then transfer it to sterilized jars.

POMADES

A pomade is a thick, rich mixture of oil and wax that has a wonderfully softening and smoothing effect on dry hands and feet. Choose carrier oils according to your skin type (see page 71). As it contains no water, a pomade can be stored for more than a month in a refrigerator.

BASIC POMADE

Essential oil
20 drops
Base
15 gm beeswax
100 ml carrier oil
4 tbsp lanolin (optional, for dry skin)

1 Measure the beeswax, carrier oil and lanolin into a heat-resistant bowl. Stir over a pan of boiling water until melted.

2 Remove the bowl from the pan. Keep stirring while the mixture begins to cool, then add the essential oil. When thickened, transfer to sterilized jars.

MASKS

Masks rejuvenate and refine the skin. I recommend deep-cleansing clay or earth masks for acne and other skin problems. They tighten as they dry, leaving skin glowing. Non-drying masks can be made from yogurt, effective for treating spots and acne, or from most fruit. AHAs (alpha hydroxy acids) in fruit have been hailed as anti-wrinkling agents: by exfoliating the skin and boosting its ability to retain water, they smooth out lines. If you are allergic to a fruit, do a patch test first: place some on your wrist, and after 30 minutes rinse with cool water. If there is a reaction, avoid.

BASIC CLAY MASK

Essential oil
1 drop
Base
1 tsp Fullers earth, kaolin
or green clay
up to 5 ml flower water or
distilled water

1 Measure the Fullers earth, kaolin or green clay into a small bowl, then stir in just enough water to make a paste.

2 Add the essential oil, and mix well. Apply the mask to clean skin, avoiding the delicate area around the eyes, and wash off thoroughly after ten minutes.

VARIATIONS

*1 **Nourishing fruit mask:** substitute avocado for fruit, add 1 tsp honey, 1 egg yolk and 2 drops lemon juice in step 1.*
*2 **Rich hair conditioner:** cover the hair with variation 1, omitting honey, leave for 30 minutes, rinse and shampoo.*
*3 **Fruit mask:** to counteract the damaging effects of the sun, use papaya with 1–2 drops orange essential oil.*
*4 **Richer drying mask:** add 2 ml jojoba to the clay mask in step 1.*

BASIC FRUIT OR
YOGURT MASK

Essential oil
1 drop
Base
1 tbsp ripe fruit or
1 tsp plain live yogurt

1 ▷ Mash the fruit and sieve it into a small bowl. If using yogurt, spoon it into the bowl.

2 Add the essential oil and mix well. Apply the mask to clean skin, avoiding the delicate area around the eyes, and wash off after ten minutes.

SIEVE THE FRUIT to create a smooth texture before adding the essential oil to the fruit mask

AROMATIC FACIAL

One of life's great luxuries, an aromatic facial with scented oil or cream improves skin tone while reducing tension and easing away worry lines. Men and women alike enjoy its delights. The massage movements stimulate the blood circulation and bring nourishment to the skin to encourage cell renewal and the elimination of waste. This truly pampering treatment leaves you feeling, and looking, years younger with glowing, healthy skin.

CLEANSING TREATMENT

Begin by applying a cleanser with smooth, gliding strokes to remove surface dirt. To relax the face and soften the skin, follow this with a hot, damp face-cloth treatment. I like to infuse a bag of peppermint tea (for oily skin) or chamomile tea (for dry or sensitive skin), or add a drop of essential oil diluted in a teaspoon of carrier oil to the hot water. The face-cloths open the pores in preparation for the massage with scented oils that follows.

SIMPLE CLEANSING OIL

Essential oils
4 drops lavender, 3 drops orange
Carrier oil
30 ml grapeseed, sunflower or soya

Follow method for Basic Oil, page 71.

LAVENDER CLEANSING CREAM

Essential oil
4 drops lavender
Base
7 gm beeswax, 60 ml sunflower oil
30 ml orange flower water

Follow method for Basic Cream, page 72.

1 Ensure your friend removes contact lenses and jewellery, and ask her to lie down on her back. Kneel behind her head and apply a cleanser with smooth, outward strokes all over the face and neck, avoiding the eyes. Remove with damp cotton wool.

2 Soak three face-cloths in a bowl of hot water containing a drop of essential oil or herbal tea bag (see above). Check the heat of the cloths, wring out and cover the face (except the nose and mouth) with two cloths. As one cools, replace it. Blot dry.

BEGINNING TO MASSAGE

GENTLE MASSAGE OIL

Essential oils
1 drop each of bergamot,
chamomile and geranium
Carrier oil
10 ml sweet almond

Follow method for Basic Oil, page 71.

JOJOBA CREAM

Essential oil
4–6 drops of either jasmine, frankincense
or lavender
Base
10 gm beeswax
25 ml sweet almond oil
20 ml sunflower oil, 35 ml jojoba
20 ml rose water or distilled water

Follow variation 1 for Basic Cream, page 72.

LUXURIOUS OIL

Essential oils
2 drops rose
1 drop each of jasmine and sandalwood
Carrier oils
5 ml each of apricot kernel and jojoba

Follow method for Basic Oil, page 71.

1 Select an aromatic oil blend or cream to suit your friend (see above), and apply a small amount to your hands to warm it. Gently place your hands on the neck and stroke up to the chin.

2 △ Swivel your hands around at the chin to sweep out toward the ears. Imagine that you are sculpting the area, giving it a face-lift as your hands mould the contours.

3 Glide back gently to the chin where your fingers touch and interlock, then stroke your hands smoothly up over the cheeks and out to the temples.

4 At the temples, swivel your hands around so that your fingers meet over the forehead, and then stroke out over the forehead to the temples. Repeat steps 1–4 at least three times.

RELEASING TENSION

1 Place the flattened fingers of both hands on the left side of the chest by the collar bone and stroke gently up to the neck at least six times. Then glide across the upper chest and repeat on the right side. If massaging a man, concentrate less on this stroking (stubble can make it uncomfortable for both of you) and more on circling and knuckling (steps 2 and 3).

2 Because so many people carry tension in the jaw, I do extra work here. Rest your left hand by your friend's left ear, and with the two middle fingers of your right hand make circles out from the chin along the left side of the jaw. Return to the chin and repeat on the right side.

3 ▷ Rotate the knuckles of both hands simultaneously on both sides of the face from under the cheek out to the jaw joints. Let each knuckle follow separately to produce a deep, steady movement.

4 With alternate hands, stroke around the chin and out along the jaw toward the ears in a rhythmic, sweeping movement. The more fluid you make this stroke, the more relaxing it will be. Repeat several times.

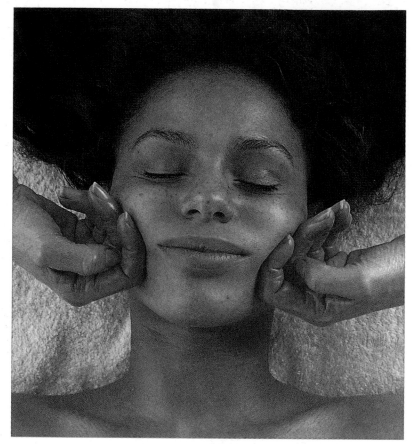

CIRCLING AWAY LINES

1 ▷ Interlock your thumbs in order to steady your hands, and with your middle fingers make circles all around the mouth and up the sides of the nose, taking care not to obstruct the nostrils. You can circle very gently or firmly — try both and ask your friend which movement she prefers.

2 Continue making circles, out from the centre of the forehead to the right temple, varying the pressure as you work. Imagine lines and wrinkles disappearing as the nourishing oils penetrate the skin, helping to improve its texture, elasticity and appearance. Repeat on the left side of the forehead.

THIS MOVEMENT, covering many acupuncture points, relieves pent-up tension

REJUVENATING THE EYES

1 Stroke your middle fingers firmly out from the bridge of the nose over the eyebrows to the temples and gently in under the eyes, making light pressures at the temples and bridge of the nose.

2 ◁ Squeeze the eyebrows between your thumbs and index fingers; hold, release and repeat, covering each brow.

3 Rest your fingers on the closed eyelids, press down very gently, then release, opening your fingers and gliding out to the temples. Repeat once. This movement can be glorious if you are sensitive to your friend: ask her if the pressure is comfortable.

RELAXING & SOOTHING

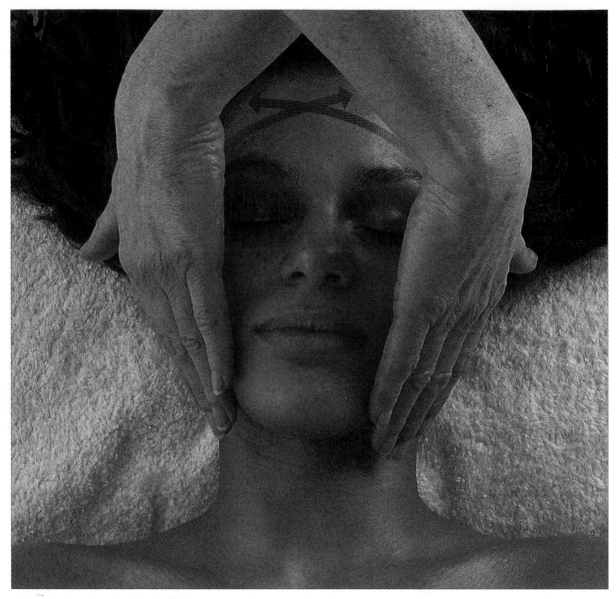

1 *Stroke up the forehead, one hand slowly following the other. The very repetitiveness of this movement is its main virtue, allowing your friend to drift away.*

2 *With your fingertips, circle gently and continuously up from the bridge of the nose to the hairline. Then separate your fingers, slide them into the hair, and gently pull large sections of hair toward you. Work all over the head. This extraordinary movement creates a sensation of floating, as the last vestiges of tension melt away.*

3 △ *Stroke your palms out from the centre of the forehead and glide down to the chin, where they cross (left hand lifts over right hand), return to the forehead and cross again. Glide your hands down the sides of the face and neck, swivel them out over the shoulders and up the back of the neck, then slide up the face to the forehead. Repeat two or three times.*

4 *Simply let your hands rest on your friend's forehead. Hold this position for at least ten seconds, and then slowly, imperceptibly, draw your hands away.*

FINAL BEAUTIFYING TOUCHES

CLAY MASK

Essential oil
1 drop of either chamomile,
geranium or orange

Base
1 tsp Fullers earth, kaolin or green clay
3 ml rose water or distilled water
2 ml jojoba (optional, for dry skin)

Follow variation 4 for Basic Clay Mask, page 73.

MILD TONER

Essential oils
10 drops each of orange and petitgrain
5 drops neroli

Base
100 ml distilled water

Follow method for Basic Toner, page 72.

GALEN'S ROSE CREAM

Essential oil
4 drops rose

Base
7 gm beeswax, 60 ml sweet almond oil
30 ml rose water or distilled water

Follow method for Basic Cream, page 72.

1 Remove the massage oil or cream with damp cotton wool, then clean your hands on a damp towel or face-cloth.

2 △ Apply a clay mask all over the face and neck, avoiding the delicate eye area. Leave the mask to dry for about ten minutes, then remove it with a warm, damp face-cloth.

3 Pour a small amount of toner on to a piece of cotton wool, and gently stroke the entire face and neck with it. This helps to freshen the skin and remove any residue of the mask.

4 With your fingers, apply the moisturizing rose cream, which prevents moisture loss and keeps the skin smooth and pliable.

NATURAL FACE-LIFT

Taking ten minutes a day to massage your face can produce amazing results— simply relaxing tired, strained muscles can leave you looking ten years younger. Although wrinkles are an inevitable part of ageing, massage can ease away microscopic lines so that your skin looks both smoother and firmer, and it can help to prevent new lines appearing too. Facial skin is delicate, so work gently using lots of scented oil that most suits your skin type (see page 71).

FOR OILY SKIN

Essential oils
2 drops bergamot
1 drop each of lemon and geranium
Carrier oil
10 ml soya

FOR SENSITIVE SKIN

Essential oils
2 drops chamomile, 1 drop lavender
Carrier oil
10 ml sweet almond

For all three recipes follow method for Basic Oil, page 71.

FOR DRY SKIN

Essential oils
2 drops neroli, 1 drop each of frankincense and rose
Carrier oils
5 ml each of sweet almond oil and jojoba

APPLYING THE OIL

Choose one of the massage oils and remove contact lenses and jewellery. Pour a small amount of the oil into your palm and warm it between your hands. Gently cup your face in your hands and after a moment slide your hands out toward your ears, drawing tension out. Repeat at least three times.

FIRMING THE NECK & CHIN

1 Open your mouth, pursing your lips tightly over your teeth to form an oval. Holding this position, make slow circular movements with the tips of your middle fingers around your mouth and chin and down to the edges of the jaw. Work up either side of the nose and out over the forehead to the temples.

2 *Flatten the fingers of your right hand and make large circles on the large muscle on the left side of the neck. Repeat using the fingers of the left hand on the right side. Then, to vary the movement, work on both sides together, using your left hand for the left side of the neck, and your right hand for the right side. Repeat around the back of the neck because tension here shows in the face.*

3 ◁ *Tilt your head to the right. Using the back of your left hand, then the back of your right hand, briskly stroke up the left side of the neck, so that one hand lifts off as the other is beginning the stroke. Repeat on the right side. These stimulating movements can help to counteract signs of ageing.*

BEAUTIFYING THE EYES

1 With your two middle fingers circle your eyes, stroking firmly out over the eyebrows and gliding very gently back under the eyes. Repeat five times.

2 Starting at the bridge of the nose, squeeze the eyebrows between your thumbs and first two fingers. Hold, and slowly release before moving on to the next area, covering the whole eyebrow.

3 Apply pressure with the middle fingers of both hands on the temples and all over the forehead. This can help relieve headaches and tension. Then use just your third fingers to apply gentle pressure along the socket bone beneath the eyes, in the direction of the nose.

4 ◁ Combat frown lines by rubbing your fingers together in a scissor-like motion across the middle of the forehead, above the eyebrows and out to each side of the forehead.

5 Slowly stroke one palm after the other from the eyebrows over the forehead and into the hair. Repeat several times.

GENTLE REVITALIZATION

1 With your fingertips, lightly tap from the chin out to the ears, then from beside the nose up to the temples and, finally, over the forehead to the temples. Tap extremely gently over the closed eyelid and beneath the eye (remove contact lenses first).

2 Enjoy the quietness and stillness of just cupping your hands over your eyes and forehead to release any last vestiges of tension. Alternatively, cup your hands over the whole face, including the chin and cheeks. Hold for several seconds.

REFRESHING FACIAL

The brisk and energetic movements in this invigorating facial massage stimulate the circulation, bringing fresh, oxygenated blood to the area and eliminating waste to leave the skin glowing. Surprisingly, vigorous strokes can be deeply relaxing and are an integral part of this particular massage. Skin toners are used to freshen the skin, remove traces of cleanser and help restore the skin's acid mantle (a fine layer that protects against infection). They can also be used after a refreshing facial to create a cooling effect. A simple splash of water is the cheapest toner, but traditional preparations also include flower waters, herbal infusions and aromatic vinegars. To preserve the natural equilibrium of the skin, I recommend mild skin fresheners.

GENTLE ROSE TONER

Essential oil
25 drops rose
Base
100 ml distilled water

Follow method for Basic Toner, page 72.

HONEY WATER

Essential oils
2 drops bergamot, 1 drop each of benzoin, sandalwood and lavender
Base
10 ml vodka
1/4 tsp honey
80 ml orange flower water

Follow method for Basic Honey Water, page 72.

AROMATIC VINEGAR

Essential oils
3 drops rosemary
2 drops rose, 1 drop lavender
Base
10 ml wine or cider vinegar
80 ml distilled water

Follow method for Basic Aromatic Vinegar, page 72.

TONING THE CHIN

1 ▷ *Choose one of the aromatic toners above and pour a small amount into your palm. Splash the toner on your face, taking care to avoid the eyes. Then, with the backs of your hands, rhythmically slap and pat the area under the chin. Repeat several times. This movement can help to combat a double chin by stimulating the circulation.*

2 Loosely roll the backs of your fingers under the chin, one hand following the other. Vary the amount of pressure from a light, vibrating movement to a firm, invigorating one. Continue on the left and right sides of the chin.

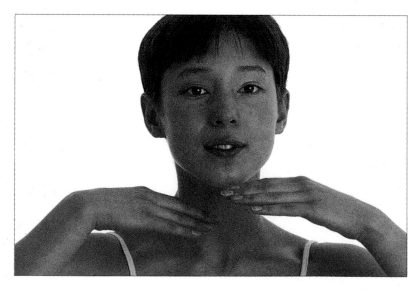

RESISTING THE EFFECTS OF AGEING

1 ◁ *Roll the skin of the right cheek with the backs of all your fingers from the side of the mouth over the cheek toward the ear. Both hands work together, one following the other. Work upward and outward, following the facial muscles to improve tone and give sagging cheeks a boost. Repeat on the left side of the face.*

2 *Ease frown lines by tapping the fleshy part of your fingers rapidly up the forehead. This percussive movement sounds like galloping horses.*

3 *Using your fingertips, lightly and rhythmically tap all over the face. Some clients say this feels like butterfly wings fluttering on the face while others claim it is like raindrops falling. On a hot day, splash some extra toner on the face and pat it in using this lovely stimulating movement to leave the skin fresh and glowing. Some men like to do this after shaving.*

INSTANT REVIVAL

1 ▷ *Starting at the bridge of your nose, make circular movements with the pads of your fingers in a straight line up to the top of your head. Then work firmly and methodically all over your head, really moving the scalp as if you were shampooing your hair. This invigorating action helps to release tension and stimulate the circulation, and can also relieve headaches.*

2 *With your fingers against the scalp, take large handfuls of hair and gently, yet firmly, pull up at the roots.*

3 *Finish the refreshing facial by using your thumbs and forefingers to massage your ears. Begin at the lobes and squeeze, rotate and release, working up to the top of the ear. Acupuncture points relating to the whole body are found on the ears and massaging these points stimulates every part of you.*

BEAUTIFYING THE BODY

Everybody should learn how to do simple self-massage as it is an excellent method of pampering yourself, and when combined with essential oils it is remarkably beneficial for areas of the body that require extra care. In just a few minutes each day, you can improve both the condition and the tone of your skin. Choose aromatic oils to suit your needs — to cleanse, stimulate or nourish — and, most importantly, ensure that you like the scent of your oil blend.

HANDS & ELBOWS

THE CONDITION OF THE HANDS and elbows depends largely on the care we give them. Age, hard work and neglect can leave them rough and dry, while water and detergents strip away protective oils. For smoother hands, massage in a nourishing cream containing a soothing oil, such as benzoin. Cover dry hands with extra rich cream at night and wear cotton gloves to bed, as did ladies of the court in Elizabethan England.

NOURISHING THE HANDS

1 Sit comfortably and apply a little cream (see opposite page) to your right palm. Stroke it on to your left hand from the fingers to the wrist. Imagine the cream penetrating the skin — relaxing, soothing and warming it. Repeat several times.

2 ▷ Supporting your left palm with the fingers of your right hand, use your thumb to stroke from the knuckle of your little finger down the tendon toward the wrist. Repeat, stroking down the tendons between each of the fingers.

3 Squeeze the base of your little finger between your thumb and forefinger and circle around either side of the finger, working up to and including the tip of the nail. Rub some cream into the cuticle and fingernail, which also benefit from pampering. Repeat on each finger and on the thumb.

4 ◁ Using the knuckles of the first and second fingers, gently grip the little finger and slowly pull it as you slide up to the tip with a corkscrew-like motion that stimulates the circulation. Repeat twice on each finger and on the thumb.

5 Support the back of the left hand with the fingers of your right hand and massage the palm with your thumb. Stroke and stretch the palm and notice tension melting away.

6 Firmly roll your middle knuckles all over the palm and finish by gently stroking the wrist, and then the hand, with your thumb. Repeat the entire sequence on the other hand.

PAMPERING THE ELBOWS

With care and attention, you can transform rough, dry and discoloured elbows. For a gentle bleaching effect, rub each elbow with half a lemon, and to reverse dryness, massage them with a generous amount of one of these rich creams, containing nourishing oils such as avocado and wheatgerm.

EXTRA RICH CREAM

Essential oil
4–6 drops of either orange or benzoin

Base
7 gm beeswax, 15 gm lanolin
30 ml sweet almond oil
15 ml wheatgerm oil
60 ml distilled water

Follow variation 2 for Basic Cream, page 72.

COCOA BUTTER CREAM

Essential oil
4–6 drops of either melissa,
rose or chamomile

Base
7 gm beeswax
15 gm cocoa butter, 20 ml avocado oil
20 ml apricot kernel oil, 5 ml carrot oil
35 ml orange flower water

Follow variation 3 for Basic Cream, page 72.

ABDOMEN, HIPS & THIGHS

MANY OF MY CLIENTS wish to transform these fleshy, untoned areas, which are prone to cellulite (dimpled flesh resembling orange peel, caused by connective tissue pulling in against the skin, making the fat bulge). Daily aromatherapy massage can improve the skin by making it appear smoother and tighter to give the illusion of lost weight. Large, firm movements boost the circulation and soft, smooth strokes stimulate the lymphatic system to help eliminate waste. Beneficial essential oils include: marjoram and peppermint to soothe the abdomen; rosemary and geranium to invigorate; and juniper to help reduce fluid retention.

SOOTHING BLEND

Essential oils
3 drops marjoram, 2 drops chamomile
1 drop peppermint
Carrier oils
18 ml sweet almond, 2 ml wheatgerm

CELLULITE BLEND

Essential oils
3 drops each of lavender and cypress
1 drop juniper
Carrier oils
18 ml sweet almond, 2 ml wheatgerm

STIMULATING BLEND

Essential oils
3 drops each of juniper and rosemary
1 drop geranium
Carrier oils
18 ml sweet almond, 2 ml wheatgerm

For all, follow method for Basic Oil, page 71.

IMPROVING THE ABDOMEN & HIPS

1 Sit comfortably and rest your left hand on your diaphragm (just under the rib cage) while your right hand applies about a teaspoon of oil with clockwise strokes around the navel (following the workings of the intestine). Now introduce the left hand to the stroke so that both hands circle the navel (see Circular Stroking, page 45). Repeat several times.

2 △ Knead the hips, waist and abdomen by squeezing and lifting the flesh with one hand and releasing it into the other. Knead all over this area, wherever you can pick up enough flesh.

3 With your left hand on top of your right, use your fingertips to apply gentle circular pressure all around the navel. Work in a clockwise direction.

4 Finish by gently stroking all over the abdomen and hips. This is very soothing and stimulates lymph drainage.

TONING THE THIGHS

1 Apply more massage oil if necessary so that your hands move smoothly over the skin. Gently stroke up from your left knee, directing your movements toward the inner thigh. Then stroke from the back of the knee up to the buttocks.

2 △ Knead the thigh from the knee up to the top of the leg. This area is fleshy, so use deep movements to squeeze and lift the flesh. These kneading strokes stimulate the circulation and break down dimpled skin by helping stored fluid and waste to be reabsorbed into the lymphatic system. Repeat on the back of the thigh.

3 ▷ Applying firm pressure, rotate the knuckles of both hands all over the front and back of the thigh.

4 Place your left hand on the back of the outer thigh, and your right hand on the back of the inner thigh. Pull the flesh up to the top of the thigh, release, and cross your hands down the other side. Repeat this criss-cross movement several times.

5 Stroke smoothly and gently from above the knee to the top of the thigh, and from the back of the knee to the buttock. This repetitive stroking encourages lymph drainage. Repeat the entire sequence on the right thigh.

THE FEET

LEONARDO DA VINCI referred to the foot as the world's greatest engineering device: it contains nearly a quarter of the body's bones and absorbs three times the body's weight with each step. Yet the feet are often neglected. Tired, aching feet affect the way you look, feel and move. Each foot contains thousands of nerve endings, and regular massage benefits the whole body while keeping the feet smooth and flexible. For a pre-massage treat, soak the feet in a basin of warm water containing four drops of essential oil: juniper, lemongrass or rosemary to combat fluid retention; cypress or geranium for cramps; or eucalyptus to revitalize.

TIRED FEET BLEND

Essential oil
4 drops of either lavender or peppermint
Carrier oil
10 ml sunflower or sweet almond

Follow method for Basic Oil, page 71.

POMADE FOR ROUGH SKIN

Essential oil
20 drops of either frankincense, geranium or sandalwood
Base
15 gm beeswax
100 ml sunflower or sweet almond oil

Follow method for Basic Pomade, page 73.

SWOLLEN FEET BLEND

Essential oils
3 drops lavender, 2 drops chamomile
Carrier oil
10 ml sunflower or sweet almond

Follow method for Basic Oil, page 71.

1 Rest your right foot on your left thigh. Support it with your right hand while your left hand strokes the sole and top of the foot from the toes up to the ankle, spreading the aromatic oil or pomade. Use your knuckles to ripple all around the sole. Then, using your thumbs, apply deep pressure to the sole of the foot (see Static Pressures, page 46). Work on the centre, outer side, and instep.

2 Massage each toe by rubbing, squeezing, and gently rolling it between your fingers. Then pinch the tip of the nail. These movements stimulate the circulation and soothe the toes.

3 Support your foot with your left hand, and clasp your toes with the right hand. Gently stretch the toes backward and forward to release tension and increase their flexibility.

4 Using your fingers, squeeze around your ankle, the Achilles tendon (directly above the heel on the back of the leg) and the heel. Then rotate your ankle several times.

5 ▷ Sandwich the foot by placing one hand on top and the other under the base of the toes, and rotate your hands around the ball of the foot to increase flexibility.

6 Finish by stroking up from the toes toward the ankle. Repeat the entire massage sequence on the left foot.

SANDWICHING AND ROLLING the foot helps to increase flexibility and release tension

SCENTED BATHING

A fragranced bath, whether warming and comforting or coolly refreshing, has always been the perfect way to shed tension. The Greek physician, Hippocrates (c.460–377BC), maintained that "the way to health is to have an aromatic bath and scented massage every day".

Most famous beauties have had extravagant bath recipes, containing ingredients such as crushed strawberries and champagne, but the simple addition of diluted essential oils can make a bath equally luxurious. If you do not have a bath, an aromatherapy shower also works wonders.

EXTRAVAGANT BLEND

Essential oils
2 drops each of neroli and rose
1 drop sandalwood
Carrier oil
5 ml sweet almond

Follow method for Basic Oil, page 71.

MILK & HONEY BATH

Essential oil
10–25 drops of mandarin or geranium
Base
1 tsp liquid detergent
110 ml of either sweet almond
or sunflower oil
25 ml vodka
55 ml milk
1 tsp honey
1 egg

*Mix the ingredients in a blender on low speed.
Makes enough for eight baths.*

WAKE-UP BLEND

Essential oils
2 drops each of petitgrain and rosemary
1 drop geranium
Carrier oil
5 ml sweet almond

Follow method for Basic Oil, page 71.

SKIN BRUSHING

◁ *Before you climb into your scented bath or step into the shower, take a few minutes to stimulate the circulation by brushing your skin with a natural fibre skin brush or glove. Use brisk, circular movements all over the body, bringing fresh blood to the surface, removing dead cells and unclogging pores.*

PREPARING THE BATH

While the bath is filling with warm water (avoid very hot water, which strips the skin of natural oils, thereby drying it out), dilute up to 5 drops of your chosen essential oils in the carrier oil. Add the oil blend when the bath is nearly full, so you can enjoy the effects fully before the oils begin to evaporate. To enhance the relaxing atmosphere, bathe by candle-light.

FRAGRANT SHOWERING

If you prefer a shower to a bath, you can still enjoy the benefits of aromatherapy by dissolving a total of 12 drops made up of three of your favourite essential oils in 30 ml liquid soap.

AFTER-CARE

1 Rub yourself briskly with a towel to dry off and stimulate the circulation.

2 ◁ Using large, circular movements, apply a generous amount of scented moisturizing cream to leave your skin feeling smooth and smelling fragrant.

NOURISHING MOISTURIZER

Essential oil
4–5 drops of marjoram
or geranium
Base
7 gm beeswax
60 ml sweet almond oil
30 ml distilled water

*Follow method for
Basic Cream, page 72.*